10 POUNDS IN 10 DAYS

10 POUNDS
IN 10 DAYS

THE SECRET CELEBRITY PROGRAMME FOR LOSING WEIGHT FAST

JACKIE WARNER

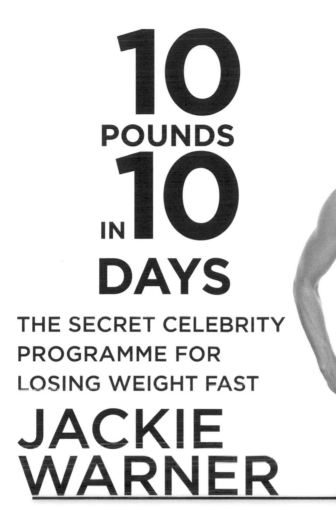

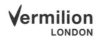

Vermilion
LONDON

10 9 8 7 6 5 4 3 2 1

Published in 2012 by Vermilion, an imprint of Ebury Publishing
First published in the USA by Grand Central Life and Style, an imprint of Grand Central Publishing, in 2012

Ebury Publishing is a Random House Group Company

The Random House Group Limited Reg. No. 954009

Addresses for companies within the Random House Group can be found at www.randomhouse.co.uk

A CIP catalogue record for this book is available from the British Library

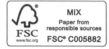

The Random House Group Limited supports The Forest Stewardship Council® (FSC®), the leading international forest certification organisation. Our books carrying the FSC label are printed on FSC® certified paper. FSC is the only forest certification scheme endorsed by the leading environmental organisations, including Greenpeace. Our paper procurement policy can be found at www.randomhouse.co.uk/environment

Printed and bound in China by Toppan
Book Design by HRoberts Design

ISBN 9780091947743

Copies are available at special rates for bulk orders. Contact the sales development team on 020 7840 8487 for more information.

To buy books by your favourite authors and register for offers, visit www.randomhouse.co.uk

Neither this diet and exercise programme nor any other diet and exercise programme should be followed without first consulting a health care professional. If you have any special conditions requiring attention, you should consult with your health care professional regularly regarding possible modification of the programme contained in this book.

Contents

Acknowledgments

Thanks so much to all those who have been so supportive of me.
I appreciate you more than you know. Mel Berger, my literary agent,
you're the best! I'm lucky to have such a great publicist and friend in
Nicole Wool. I don't know what I would do without my valued team,
Ashley Conrad and Lisa and Nina Kovner. I'm so excited to continue
working with you and to see what the future brings. Most of all, thank
you to my supporters, fans, and clients who have always been such a
bright light in my life. I love what I do and I love doing it for you.

Making a positive

change in your body

WILL change your

energy and open doors.

Each small step forward

leads you to endless life

possibilities.

With love,

Jackie Warner

Introduction

The Power of 10

SINCE THE RELEASE OF MY FIRST BOOK, *This Is Why You're Fat*, I've received so much feedback from my readers. In fact, people approach me now more than they ever did in response to my TV shows, Bravo's *Workout* and *Thintervention*. They're excited because they got amazing results—an average weight loss of 4–5lb (1.8–2.2kg) a week the first month of my program, right on down to their goal.

That is a very healthy pace to lose weight! But I'd be lying if I said that's the *only* healthy way to do it. There is another way: my 10x10 Program, in which you can lose 10lb (4.5kg) in ten days. That's what this book is all about.

My 10x10 Program is so successful, I decided that losing weight fast and healthily shouldn't be reserved for the entertainment elite or for those who can afford to come and see me. It is possible for anyone to achieve fast results in ten days or even more amazing results with my 30-day program if you're ready to get focused and change your life!

The Inspiration

To say that proper nutrition and exercise changed who I am is an understatement. Growing up, I was actually very shy. I was the student and athlete who coasted through life and did the bare minimum to get by. None of this was very good for my self-esteem, by the way. I so wish I'd known back then that I was causing my own misery through the food choices I was making.

When I was 18, I moved from my small midwestern Christian town to Los Angeles to go to college. In only about four months, I blew up from 8st 4lb to 12st 1lb (52.5kg to 76.5kg). I was lonely; I knew no one, and this caused me to self-medicate with fast food. The fatter I got, the shyer I got. My confidence plummeted.

One day, I was sitting in my dorm room, looking in the mirror, and I started crying. I knew deep down I would never succeed if I continued to feel this way about myself and to present a damaged self-image to the world.

That very day, I decided to do something about my misery. I stopped eating fast food. I started walking to and from college—a total of 40 blocks a day. The weight fell off, and I couldn't wait to learn more. I started going to the gym and reading books about whole foods and nutrition.

The more I set and kept goals and the better I felt, the more type-A I became. I started to look directly into people's eyes when talking to them. I spoke with more authority. My whole energy changed.

This isn't just me talking, either. It's been proven in research: when people make positive changes in body composition, strength, and endurance, their entire self-worth almost always improves.

I've lived it and I've dedicated my life's work to helping others find a way to a fit life that brings happiness, worthiness, and health.

If it weren't for this experience, I would not be sharing with you today the knowledge I've cultivated over the past 20 years. I want you to join me in creating the life you deserve, and the best-looking body possible.

All you need to do is what I did: make the decision to live differently. It's not easy, but nothing worth having ever is. I promise that when you commit to my new 10x10 Program, you'll experience change like you've never felt before, and experience success you never thought possible.

The Creation

A little background: a year ago, I was going through many of the old programs, graphics, and ideas that I have had since I became certified 15 years ago. It was particularly fun looking at all the stuff from my first gym, Lift in Beverly Hills. I rolled up on a two-page diet called "Lose 10lbs in 10 days." So obviously, this is not a new concept that is just now catching fire. This was—and is—what people *really* want, and I was addressing that desire even back then.

I found that with women in particular, if I couldn't get them to drop two sizes in two weeks, they would get frustrated, start sabotaging themselves, and fall off the plan. My old program was pretty severe: egg whites, a can of plain tuna, celery, fish, and broccoli; in keeping with the times, I also pushed fat-free desserts. The program didn't address how to lose additional weight or how to maintain your new body. Let me apologize now to all of my old clients: what a slice of hell that was to follow!

Since then, I've modified and refined that plan, based on more years of experience and data from the most cutting-edge researchers working with me. After all the heavy research, I test every component of a program on men and women of all backgrounds and with different goal weights, as well as with my celebrity clients, to get real-life results. I then tweak accordingly. That's the careful process that goes into all of my work.

The result is that now I can give you a nutrient-rich, easy-to-follow program that your body will love and that you will commit to for a lifetime. It helps you take off 10lb (4.5kg) in ten days, and lets you continue your weight loss for the next 20 days—a full 30 days of fat burning and body toning.

My 10x10 Program is powerful and designed to:

√ *Change your body chemistry in a day*

√ *Change the genes you were born with*

√ *Change your set point*

√ *Change your relationship with food*

The Motivation

Fast Is Safe and Better

I have honed this fast and effective diet throughout the years because there was such a demand from my clients. Some of my personal clients and members of my world-renowned gyms who have benefited from this program and other Jackie Warner programs include: Julia Roberts, Paul McCartney, Heather Mills, Anne Hathaway, Alanis Morissette, Eve, Kathy Griffin, Maria Shriver, America Ferrera, Amber Tamblyn, Amanda Peet, Giuliana Rancic, Kerry Washington, James Van Der Beek, Adam

Goldberg, Hal Sparks, Jody Watley, and Nia Vardalos.

Celebrities are unique because losing weight post-baby or getting red-carpet-ready becomes a national media event. They typically call me and say, "I have two weeks to get into my gown for the Oscars," or "I have to show my half-naked body for my upcoming movie." No pressure there! That's why my celebrity clients love my 10x10 Program: because they always need to get their bodies in great shape in a short time.

The 10x10 Program offers a detailed plan, grocery lists, workouts, and tools. With this program, you're setting yourself on the path toward living the fittest, happiest, and healthiest life possible.

One of the benefits of the 10x10 Program is that it's broken down into three 10-day phases and organized so you don't have to think about what you need to do. From meals to exercise sessions to motivational support, the 10x10 Program has everything you need to kick-start your new life of fitness, health, and happiness!

You will lose up to 10lb (4.5kg) in the first ten days if you follow the 10x10 Program exactly as written. It's worked for my celebrity clients, it's worked for my other clients, and it's worked for me. You only have to commit to each ten-day phase until you achieve your personal weight-loss, nutrition, and fitness goals. I promise, you'll see yourself, and the world, differently.

Jackie's Total Support System

I want you to know that you can succeed no matter where you live, and no matter what your circumstances or background. I changed my life completely by applying three simple rules for success, and now I have created the steps for you to do the same. You cannot change the outer body without changing your inner chemistry. The only way to do this is to:

√ **Eat**—*Eat a nutrient-rich, all-natural diet.*

√ **Move**—*Commit to intensive and consistent workouts.*

√ **Believe**—*Create strong psychological tools to help reframe your thinking.*

Without these steps, tackling weight issues and experiencing a happy, healthy lifestyle are extremely difficult. Why? Because your body is out of balance, and it's only the adoption of this philosophy that can change your body chemistry and set you on the path to true health. In this book, I will teach you how to eat, move, and believe your way to the life that you deserve.

Let me explain . . .

Eat: Free Yourself from Old Beliefs About Food

Convenience is killing us. Fast food and processed foods may make our lives easier, but the problems they've introduced into our society are making us sick and fat.

Don't rely on the food industry to take care of you. They only care about profit. I will share with you all-natural chemistry-balancing foods that jump-start your metabolism, turning your body into a fat-burning machine. You'll lose weight and gain back your health.

Move: It's Time to Free Your Body to Be the Best It Can Be

Human beings are designed to move. Unfortunately, contemporary lifestyles and the conveniences brought on by technology have turned many people into rather sedentary beings.

Instead of getting up to change the TV channel, we use a remote control. Instead of participating in sports, we play tennis, football, baseball, basketball, dance, and any other sport we like on Xbox, Wii, and PlayStation.

Without movement, we slow ourselves down—literally! Our bodies need to move to function at their best. The 10x10 Program gets you moving, and in the process helps your body return to its natural state: that of **fitness, strength, and balance**.

Believe: Free Your Mind from Negative Self-Talk

Did you know that negative self-talk can actually create neural connections in the brain that perpetuate an unhealthy state? The bad stuff you think about yourself can cause a chemical change in your body that makes it harder to lose weight. I'm going to give you the tools to change your self-loathing into self-loving.

Ignite the Inner Fire!

I am so excited to think about the amazing changes you are about to make. You've tried diets that didn't work. You've done workouts that didn't deliver. You've pushed yourself into a corner because you're so overscheduled that making more time to make more thoughtful, nutritious choices seems impossible. I want you to know that you can succeed no matter what. I changed my life completely by applying these three simple rules. I'm here to share with you that not only is a healthy lifestyle possible; it is the only way to live! The 10x10 Program will ignite that inner fire!

PART 1

Lose 10 Pounds in 10 Days

THE OVERRIDING REASON WHY

10x10 works so well is because it's research-backed and client-proven. The fascinating research I will share with you supports what I see in my gyms and with my clients every single day. The wonderful feedback I've received on the 10x10 Program is that not only do people lose 10lb (4.5kg), but they feel energized doing it. I don't want to create a bunch of skinny, bitchy, miserable people. My number one goal in life is to help people go from unhappy to happy. And that is how you will start feeling when you take control of your health and your weight.

My career as a wellness professional has been so successful mainly because I love to study human nature. I'm fascinated by what drives people to fail and to succeed.

Here's what makes you fail:

👎 You don't feel your body image or energy is negatively affected enough to do the hard work it takes to look and feel better.

👎 You follow complicated diets or exercise programs that cause your brain to become either distracted or filled with info that leads you to quit.

👎 You feel your goal is unreachable and the work you're doing just isn't worth the results you're seeing.

👎 You keep following diet and exercise fads that are trying to sell a different principle (stability training or ab machine workouts) instead of the *best* principles.

👎 And finally, the article or book or infomercial tip you heard gives you *way* too many choices, confusing your decision-making process.

My program overcomes all these obstacles and gets you excited about the fast results you will experience. Here's why you *will* succeed on 10x10:

👍 The diet is so simple, your brain doesn't even need to think.

👍 The exercises can be done anytime, anywhere, whether you're at home, at the gym, or in a hotel room (if you're on vacation or travel for work).

👍 The goal is set for you, and if you follow the basic steps you will reach it.

👍 The principles are the *best* way to lose weight, not the next fad that won't stick.

👍 The decisions are made for you. There are no substitutions and there's no way to talk yourself into cheating.

The next three chapters will give an overview of what's essential to any successful weight-loss program. It's organized in the Jackie Warner philosophy that you Eat + Move + Believe to have lasting results.

Eat + Move + Believe

- ☐ a simple and super effective diet

- ☐ to go from a fat-storing machine to a fat-burning machine fast

- ☐ how to turn off bad genes and turn on the good ones

- ☐ what your set point is and how to change it

- ☐ how to get maximum results from your workouts in minimum time

- ☐ cutting-edge training techniques like cardio-acceleration

- ☐ which goals to set and how to achieve them

- ☐ how to turn self-loathing into self-loving and achieve your dreams

Basically, if you know anything about me from television, my countless interviews, and my previous book, you know that I cut through all that BS and give you principles that really work. I don't just want you to get a six-pack. I really want you to fall in love with your body. I deal with the whole person and want you to have a balanced and happy life. You will succeed on this program, just as thousands of my clients have.

CHAPTER 1

Why 10x10 Really Works

I'VE TRIED EVERY DIET OUT THERE ON MYSELF. I remember trying the Atkins diet when it came out. Let me tell you, I was a monster to be around. I felt so deprived and toxic that I couldn't even think straight. It is very important that any food program makes you feel good and balanced. The 10x10 Program will do that.

You're about to find out just how simple and doable 10x10 is. I've created the easiest-to-follow diet that you will ever find. There are no recipes, either. Outside of slapping two slices of bread together or sticking a chicken breast in the oven, you can go to the grocery store and buy everything you need—already prepared. I have literally taken all the thinking out of this plan by giving you your ten-day grocery list. In short, I'll be making the decisions for you, so just get excited and go for the ride!

Depending on your weight-loss goals, either you will be following a ten-day diet (at 950 calories) for a ten-pound weight loss, or you can go all the way with the 20-day diet (at 1,200 calories) or a 30-day diet (at 1,500 calories). It is up to you how far you want to go and how much you want to lose. I designed a companion exercise program for each ten days that is perfect for what your goal will be.

So each ten days you will have a calorie adjustment, new foods, and a new workout program designed to keep you losing fat, gaining muscle, and feeling energized. It is so easy—really a no-brainer to stick to. Why? Because you'll eat the same foods each day for ten whole days, then switch to the next menu for the next ten days.

The diet is balanced and nutrient-rich with "superstar foods" that research has shown have the most fat-burning, muscle-building, and mood-stabilizing bang for their buck.

Whether you want to lose 10lb or 50lb (4.5kg or 22.5kg), my graduated calorie plans help your body continue to get balanced and bring you to your ideal weight. At the end of the 30 days, I'll put you on a plateau-busting maintenance program with fun foods and exercise combos that are designed to help you keep off the weight and adjust your body to your new healthy lifestyle.

Here's an overview of how and why my 10x10 Program works so effectively.

Built-In Goal Setting

Most people get into trouble when they don't have clear goals for getting healthy and in shape. Or the goals they do have are unrealistic and don't fit into their life. Unrealistic can mean either the goal is too big to be achieved quickly or it isn't a goal they are committed to 100 percent.

If you are five-foot-two with a mesomorph body (stocky or muscular frame), don't pull out a picture of Giselle and dream of having her ecto-morph body (lean). Focus on what's realistic for you, such as your weight before you got heavy or, if you have always been heavy, your ideal weight as charted for you in this book.

You may have read the book *The Secret*. It's a book that talks about harnessing positive energy to manifest the destiny that you dream of. The tool that is used is called a visualization board; there you write down or put up pictures of your goals to focus on daily. This is not a new concept, but it's a very sound one that will really help you to actualize your dreams. These are the steps to setting your goals:

1. Get a journal and define not only your weight-loss goal but your health goal, too.

2. Write down exactly how you would like to feel about yourself and how your life will improve as you achieve your goal.

3. Write three *very* easy things you can realistically do to reach your goal.

4. Visit your journal frequently (preferably before bed each night), writing down your feelings and thoughts about yourself. Be as gentle and positive as a therapist would be.

5. Post a picture prominently of yourself at your dream weight or a similar body type.

Goal setting starts with a clear definition of something you know you are capable of doing. Do not set a goal that doesn't fit into your lifestyle. For example, I hate to cook but I wanted to try a food program that required it. Yeah, that lasted about two weeks. I wasn't choosing a diet that worked with my busy lifestyle. Humans run from complications or stressors, so stop setting up those roadblocks.

Also, you must set up your environment for change. What have *you* changed today in order to help you reach your goal that made it impossible in the past?

Next, every time your brain tries to talk you out of your goal, shut it down and clearly state your goal followed by these words: "I will do it."

Lastly, at the end of each day, link a positive reward to a day well done.

Here is an example of how a simple goal should be achieved and supported. Let's start with water, the most powerful weight-loss and beautifying tool in your arsenal:

GOAL:

✔ Drink two to three liters of water a day. (Three liters speeds up your metabolism by about 33 percent.)

SUPPORT STEPS:

✔ Buy and keep stocked one-liter containers of water or one-liter reusable bottles and fill them two or three times throughout the day.

✔ Make drinking water as important as brushing your teeth. Leave yourself little reminders.

✔ Reward yourself by doing something relaxing and enjoyable at the end of the day, like taking a bath or drinking your favorite tea.

It's also very important to create goals beyond just weight loss. My most successful clients are the ones who link success to feeling better or sleeping better, in general being healthier. Set three goals that you can achieve on a regular basis. It may seem simple, but it's an incredibly effective way to build your self-worth and your sense of accomplishment. The act of succeeding on a daily basis will make you feel wonderful about yourself.

SET EASY GOALS

☐ Go online and search for a new fitness class in your area that you've always wanted to try, like Muay Thai (a combat sport from Thailand) or mat Pilates.

☐ Learn a new healthy recipe.

☐ Be active for 20 minutes each day even if it's just running around your block ten times.

☐ Try a new fruit or vegetable.

☐ Switch to organic foods.

☐ Replace factory-farmed meats and dairy with free-range and hormone-free meats and dairy.

☐ Enter a race for a charity. It doesn't matter if you walk or run. It matters that you do it.

Taking any one of these actions will set you forward and on your way to a new, healthy life.

The Power of Fast Weight Loss

All great trainers find a speciality that they consistently work to perfect throughout their careers. Mine is quick and lasting weight loss. I know what you're thinking: *Do I have to starve myself down to size?*

No! If you go on a starvation-type diet, your brain says *Enough!* and adjusts your metabolism to a crawl in order to stop muscle and tissue wasting. My diet does initially restrict calories but does not cause muscle wasting because every day you will be feeding your body highly nutrient superstar foods that your body has been starving for! We have been told our whole lives: If we lose weight fast, we put it back on just as fast. False! The latest research into weight loss has found that people who lose weight rapidly at the beginning of a program are so motivated by their results, not only do they stick to the diet better, but more important, *they keep the weight off longer*.

Why is this?

First, motivation. Beginning any diet is hard, but once you see the results, you want to keep going. Patients on gradual-loss diets get disheartened and want to quit. There is a strong psychological component to fast weight loss, in other words. When you see the numbers on the scale going down every single day, you get excited and want to stick with the program. The trouble with slow diets is you tend to feel you are getting nowhere and give up. Fast results keep you motivated and feeling like you are making progress.

Second, appetite. Rapid weight loss reduces your appetite along with reducing your excess weight. There is good evidence that faster weight loss triggers ketogenesis—the release of ketones into the body when fat is broken down for energy. Ketones, which are molecules of oxygen and carbon formed during fat burning, activate the release of cholecystokinin (CCK), a powerful anti-hunger hormone. CCK helps regulate your satiety, the feeling of fullness that stops hunger. By increasing feelings of fullness or satiation,

CCK keeps your appetite and cravings in check. Basically, when you're on a fast weight-loss program, you're not really hungry.

So put aside what you've heard about quick weight loss. My research shows it is the very best way if it's done right.

Rapid Weight Loss Curbs Your Appetite

Researchers from the University of Florida found that, of 262 overweight women, those who lost weight the fastest lost more and kept it off longer than those who opted for slow and steady weight loss.

Low Calorie Works!

Low-calorie diets are healthy if you follow the guidelines ensuring that your body gets what it needs to function. For example:

- Initially, calories should be low enough to cause ongoing fat loss, with a slight progressive increase to enhance metabolism.
- Eat five meals a day, consumed every two to three hours to prevent insulin drops, sluggish metabolism, and cravings.
- Choose foods with high nutrient values to sustain your energy throughout the day.

In my last book, *This Is Why You're Fat*, I told you that there are three culprits making Westerners fat:

- Imbalanced hormones
- Toxic organs
- Sugar addiction

And that's true; they factor in greatly. But losing weight is most influenced by calories in, calories out. This means that through body functions and daily movement, you have to burn more calories than you take in if you want to lose fat. You need to either work out to burn 500 calories a day or decrease your food calories by 500 to lose just one pound per week. This should drive home the importance of decreased calories and increased workouts during each phase of the 10x10 Program. When you reduce calorie intake by altering your diet, and increase calorie burning through physical activity, your body starts to burn fat, and your weight reduces. Although low in calories, this diet is balanced and nutrient-rich with Superstar Foods that change your body chemistry immediately as well as turning bad genes into good ones!

I found so much research to support low-calorie diets that I could have turned that into a book! The best way to lose weight and keep off the pounds is to do it quickly, and with greatly reduced calories.

Remember, you are staying at 950 calories for only ten days. You can look forward to increases as you go. The key here is trusting that you are accessing a very well-designed diet plan that includes all the nutrients your body needs to achieve a healthy and happy lifestyle.

900 Is the Magic Number

A University of Kentucky study indicates that people who eat no more than 900 calories a day are more likely to keep the pounds off than those on higher-calorie plans. The study involved 112 patients at the university's Weight Management Program. Participants lost an average of 4st 9lb (30kg) over five months and maintained a good percentage of their weight loss after five years.

The Balanced Diet

Balance is defined as "bringing elements into harmony." If you think of the term *elements* as "food" and *harmony* as "a healthy body," then there is a truly balanced diet out there that the body works best with and will respond to greatly. Just as your car engine requires gas, oil, and electricity to run, the body requires fat, carbs, and protein to function properly. Carbs, protein, and fat used in the right proportions are what your body craves in order to be a fat-burning machine. My diet features a 45–35–20 ratio, meaning 45 percent carbohydrates, 35 percent protein, and 20 percent fat from total daily calorie intake. Science and success tell us that the body functions optimally with this type of food intake. But don't worry: You don't have to do any math to figure out those ratios. It drives me crazy when books and magazines act as if you have nothing better to do than calculate your proteins each day and weigh out your portions. I always say that if you're forced to overthink a weight-loss program, you are more likely to fail. I'm going to make it easy for you and just tell you what the ratio of optimal eating is, then give you the easiest way to measure portion size when you start my program. This is the only way that I do it for myself and my clients. Most of us have a hard time knowing how much a gram or an ounce weighs, so I will simplify it even further for you.

I'm always blown away by how little people know and how much is misunderstood about carbs, protein, and fat. I can only blame the food industry's greed and so-called experts that are trying to profit off fad diets for misleading the public about carbs and fat in particular. So first, a little nutrition 101.

What Is a Carb?

Just like fats, carbs have been made out to be the bad guy. The carb that you have learned to be terrified of is bread in any form. I wish I had a dollar for every woman who has told me she doesn't eat carbs because she doesn't eat bread. When I dig further, these women usually tell me they eat some fruit, veggies, and beans. So guess what? Those are carbs!

The fact is, carbohydrates make up the largest portion of the best fat-burning diets. Carbohydrates are muscle and brain fuel. They are not your enemy, and they will make you thin—not fat—if eaten in the right ratio. Of course, you must choose the best carbohydrates, such as fruits, veggies, and grains high in fiber and rich in nutrients.

There are two types of carbs: fast digesting and slow digesting. Slow-digesting carbs are the preferred carbs for weight loss.

Slow-digesting carbs are natural. You'll find them in yams, brown or wild rice, red potatoes, fruit, and beans. I explained in *This Is Why You're Fat* that insulin spikes can make you gain weight. Slow-digesting carbs slow down insulin levels, which means that blood sugars remain relatively normal.

Fast-digesting carbs are man-made. They are found in breads (including bagels, buns, and rolls), white rice, cold cereals, rice cakes, and fruit juices. Think of it this way: Avoid carbs that are processed in any way, such as those included in pre-prepared items. Fast-digesting carbs can increase blood sugar levels, which releases insulin, which can make you gain weight.

If you eat a slow-digesting fruit right after your workout, the sugar in that fruit rushes to muscles to help them replenish lost glycogen, the fuel your muscle runs on. Your body is reenergized and repaired so you can maintain that beautiful muscle tone. Having muscle tone is so important for weight loss because it speeds up your metabolism greatly, even as you sleep. Starchy carbs are super-loaded with fiber, which dilutes toxic agents in the bowel, controls appetite, and moves fat out of your body before it has time to get stored.

If your diet is too low in carbs, you feel tired, moody, or obsessive about food, or have difficulty concentrating. Your body will be soft and untoned because you won't be able to build muscle and shape properly. All my friends know (because I don't shut up about it) that I have a hard time maintaining muscle. I can get very "skinny fat," to the point of unattractively gaunt. That's because I slip on my diet occasionally and don't eat enough carbs with my proteins. The trick is eating the right kind of both types of carbs in the right food combinations. I have balanced the 10x10 Program with this in mind completely.

What Is a Protein?

Now on to protein. Protein helps curb your appetite, has a direct fat-burning and hormone-balancing effect, helps relieve anxiety, and builds and maintains muscle so that even a ten-minute workout is not wasted. It's best to eat protein throughout the day, at each meal, even in snacks.

Proteins are made up of long chains of amino acids. There are 22 different types of amino acids, and the body needs all of them to function properly. There are many forms of protein, which all play an important role in the function of the body. For example, collagen is a protein of the skin; the more you replenish it, the younger and more beautiful you look.

After clients have been on my diet for just one week, I notice a big difference in their skin. It's even-toned, clear, and smooth. So, since I am obsessed with naturally turning back the clock, protein is a must.

When the proteins that we consume in our foods are broken down through digestion into individual amino acids, these amino acids are absorbed and re-formed in order to create new proteins, which are then used by the body.

Protein is found in foods such as meat, poultry, seafood, dairy foods, eggs, nuts/seeds, and legumes like lentils, chickpeas, and black beans.

You can usually tell when people don't have enough protein in their diet just by looking at them. One of my favorite markets in LA specializes in vegan and raw foods. You'd think the customers would all look vibrant, energetic, and healthy, but they don't. Many of them look emaciated and have a bluish gray tone to their skin. It's because they don't get enough protein in their diets, and their bodies show it. I've been a vegan, so I know there's a way to live this lifestyle and be healthy, but clearly a lot of people don't.

The body *must have protein* to function properly at the most basic level. That's why I'm such a strong advocate for making sure people get enough protein in their diet. It's not just a good idea—it's absolutely essential for the body to work properly and to be healthy.

If you miss a source of protein in your meals, you may feel highs and lows in your energy and be hungry more often. If your diet is too low in protein, you may find that you get sick more and lack muscle tone. Remember, the more muscle you have on your body, the faster your metabolism. Foods promote health and weight loss, but muscles turn you into a fat-burning machine.

What Is a Fat?

We can all now see where the fat-free craze of the 1980s and '90s got us . . . fatter and sicker than ever. As the food industry was creating fat-free "weight-loss" products, they took fats out but then had to add flavor by putting sugar in. Sugar, not fat, is actually the leading cause of weight gain. Fats are long-range fuel sources that supply beneficial fat-soluble vitamins, which nonfat foods lack. By eating foods lower in fat, but higher in sugar, we all got fatter.

Fats are broken down during digestion into individual fats like the polyunsaturated, monounsaturated, saturated, and trans fats. Fat is necessary for multiple body functions like production of bile and hormones, insulation of organs, and absorption of vitamins. If you eat more fat than you need for these basic functions, off it goes to storage.

Eliminating all fat from a diet is unhealthy. Here's what you want to avoid:

- High-fat snack foods, especially those with saturated or trans fats
- Fast-food/restaurant meals
- Foods with added butter, margarine, mayo, or oil (except olive oil)
- Fatty meats and dairy like bacon, rib-eye steaks, cheese made from cow's milk, and butter

Basically, these are all the foods I grew up on in Ohio! Fast food and Doritos were a huge part of my life back then, and I am certain that as a teen I was rotten inside.

Simple = Success

Remember, *you* are in charge of your body and your progress. I'm not going to be there to measure out your food portions, make sure you're doing intense workouts, or ambush you on margarita Mondays. But trust me to do most of the thinking for you. That's all I ask. If you try to overthink this, you may make bad decisions—say, crowding foods into one part of the day, or changing ingredients. Every part of this program has been well thought out; there's a definite rhyme and reason to it. You'll eat first thing in the morning, then wait two and a half hours after each meal or snack to keep your metabolism charged. And remember, you'll be eating

Foods Highest in Fat-Soluble Vitamins

One of the most important functions of fat is that it helps the body absorb fat-soluble vitamins. I've listed them below, along with their food sources you find on my diet.

VITAMIN A	VITAMIN D	VITAMIN E	VITAMIN K
Sweet potatoes	Salmon	Almonds	Herbs (dried and fresh)
Carrots	Eggs	Avocados	Dark leafy greens
Dark leafy greens	Mushrooms	Pine nuts	Onions
Red-leaf lettuce		Dried herbs (basil and oregano)	Broccoli
		Cooked spinach	Chili powder, curry powder, paprika, and cayenne
		Walnuts	Asparagus
			Cucumbers

specific fat-burning foods, and exercising with fat-burning moves. Follow the 10x10 Program to the letter, and you'll be 10lb (4.5kg) lighter at the end of the first ten days. Knowing that you will eat the same thing every day is psychologically comforting. I understand very well the complex sabotage mechanisms we all have devised for ourselves. That's exactly why I made the 10x10 Program so simple—so you could *not* have any excuses!

Let's Get Going

If you're anything like me, you want to know not only what to do to lose weight and keep it off, but *why* you are doing it. Along the way, I'm going to show you really fun and interesting facts about what the foods and exercises I give you do to your body.

Remember, after the first ten days, if you want to lose more than 10lb (4.5kg), you simply graduate to the 30-day program outlined in this book to get down to your ideal weight. You can continue to lose about 4–5lb (1.8–2.2kg) per week, depending on your goals and the size at which you start the 10x10 Program.

I have said in many interviews that any good trainer can get 10lb (4.5kg) off a client—but few clients can keep it off. I've gone a long way to solve that problem by designing a healthy, rapid weight-loss program that will inspire you to take it all off, right down to your goal. You'll light that inner fire that comes from seeing fast results.

CHAPTER 2

The Truth About Your Metabolism

AS YOU PROGRESS THROUGH MY PROGRAM, you will manipulate calories through diet and exercise to take off 10lb (4.5kg) initially, then the rest of your weight afterward. But there's more to it than that. You will be manipulating other aspects of weight loss, too. I call them **the Five Truths About Your Metabolism**:

1. Your genes

2. Your set point

3. Your biochemistry

4. Your sleep cycles

5. Your thought process

Your Genes: How to Change Your Genetic Shape

You are born with a set DNA. Some genes are dictators. The genes for your eye color or hair color, for example, issue strict orders. If they call for you to have blue eyes or brown hair, that's it. But the genes for weight are different. They are more like consultants giving suggestions. You can negotiate, and sometimes even reject, what they have in mind for you by the foods you choose and the way you live.

Many of us need only look at our parents and grandparents to know what we're working with or against. For instance, if I didn't watch my diet, and exercise, I would have a wide, flat butt and sloping shoulders. (Sorry, Mom!) We used to think that we're born with fixed genes and cannot change them too much. The most exciting research to come out now indicates that not only can genes change, but they can be activated or turned off with different foods and exercise.

Change Your Diet, Change Your Genes—and Your Jeans!

Scientists from the Netherlands reported that consuming a certain dairy drink containing probiotics changed the activity of hundreds of genes in the small intestine that control the immune system. And researchers from Baylor University (Waco, Texas) showed that a combination of whey protein (which is on my diet) and other nutrients activated genes that control lean muscle mass.

Most of us think of our genes as more or less locked in our bodies, waiting to be passed on to future generations. But your genes at every moment are very active. They are interacting with your environment. They are interacting with every bite of food you take. They are interacting with your thoughts and your feelings. When you eat food, literally, the information—beyond the food's calories—goes right into your cells and switches genes on or turns them off. The whole food-to-gene process is called nutrigenomics, and my diet is based on it.

Not to pick on my mom, but she had a full hysterectomy, fibromyalgia, foot problems resulting in painful surgery, depression, and heart problems resulting in meds and cancer—all before she reached the age I am now. My grandmother did not fare much better, suffering with psoriasis and a variety of mental disorders. So I don't exactly come from good breeding, but I have drastically changed my genes for the better with food and exercise.

If you're wondering how genes make you skinny or fat, let me elaborate. If you drink a cola, it breaks down to pure sugar, or glucose, which goes straight to your bloodstream. At the molecular level, the sugar interacts with genes by binding to proteins called transcription factors, which regulate gene expression, meaning the way genes are switched on and off. Sugar will switch on genes that tell the body to store fat—in other words, it turns on messages that make you gain weight. But if your diet is full of fiber and whole foods with the equivalent amount of calories, it has a different effect. It switches on genes that tell your body to burn fat. Or if you eat some lean protein at every meal, that meal's calories will be released more slowly into your bloodstream, and you won't get hungry.

The same goes for fat. Most people don't realize that the trans fats found in processed foods turn on messages that add weight, slow our metabolism, and cause inflammation, which can make it more likely that we'll get diabetes and other diseases. It's a pretty vicious process, wouldn't you agree? But if we eat the right fats—like omega-3 fat from fish oil, flaxseed, walnuts, and salmon—they will activate the genes that help us lose weight and get healthier.

Some companies are marketing nutrigenomic diets on the Internet and charging $2,000 or more for a genetic test and a personalized diet plan claiming to counter your genetic predisposition to obesity and many diseases. In my 10x10 Program, I have chosen the best foods to turn on your best genes! Foods that alter genes positively include brightly colored vegetables, blueberries, salmon, walnuts, olive oil, and watercress—all of which are on my diet.

My 10x10 Program focuses on foods that switch off fat genes and send the body fat-burning messages. It gives you an easy-to-follow diet that shows you exactly which foods "talk" to your genes and trigger weight loss, health, and energy. With this approach, you'll get everything you need to immediately put yourself on the path to feeling and looking better.

So just remember: Certain foods can greatly help give you a beautiful, toned body—even if you've inherited a tendency to be chubby and unhealthy. When you eat them daily, you will feel and look better daily.

Your Set Point and How to Reset It

Do you ever wonder why it's so hard to lose weight and keep it off after going on a diet? Well, one huge factor is that you may be trying to go under your body's natural "set point."

Set point is the weight that your body wants to be. As for what determines your set point in the first place, it's roughly influenced 40 percent by genetics and 60 percent by environment. If you look at your biological family, you get an idea of where your weight's set point is. The environmental factors include weight gain after pregnancy; poor nutrition; lack of exercise; stressful life-changing events, such as a lost job; or certain prescription drugs, such as antidepressants and steroids. So now you know the unfortunate truth that your body will fight you forever if you try to stay under your set weight. This is why dieting usually works for three months as opposed to three years.

I read a very interesting article that said American women's true set point was closer to the ideal woman's weight of the 1950s. Marilyn Monroe, for example, was about 8st 13lb to 10st (56.5 to 63.5kg) at her heaviest and she was only 5ft 5½ inches (166cm) tall. By today's unrealistic standards, that's considered heavy, even though those curves are really the ideal.

Experts say you can deduce your own set point by thinking back to your weight when you hit puberty, then increasing it by roughly 10lb (4.5kg). I was 8st 6lb (53kg) at puberty, and now my set point stays between 9st 4lb and 9st 9lb (59 and 61kg).

If you had a childhood weight problem, it's a little more challenging to figure out your set point. But one way you can do it is to look at the ideal weight ranges in the tables below. They're determined through a very simple calculation: The lower end of the range is for small-boned individuals; the upper end, for larger-boned people.

I know from my experience that women in particular have a distorted body image. Some of you who buy this book really don't need to lose weight but just want to be as skinny as possible. Some of you may need only to lose close to 10lb (4.5kg). And some of you have serious weight-loss goals.

Having an unrealistic idea of your set point will only cause pain and frustration. So figure out your best goal weight by considering your set point and considering the information in the charts. Write down your goal weight.

Women

SMALL-BONED FRAME			MIDPOINT			LARGE-BONED FRAME		
5' (152cm)	=	6st 1lb (38.5kg)	5' (152cm)	=	7st 2lb (45.3kg)	5' (152cm)	=	8st 3lb (52.1kg)
5'1" (155cm)	=	6st 6lb (40.8kg)	5'1" (155cm)	=	7st 7lb (47.6kg)	5'1" (155cm)	=	8st 9lb (54.8kg)
5'2" (157cm)	=	6st 10lb (42.6kg)	5'2" (157cm)	=	7st 12lb (49.8kg)	5'2" (157cm)	=	9st 1lb (57.6kg)
5'3" (160cm)	=	7st (44.4kg)	5'3" (160cm)	=	8st 3lb (52kg)	5'3" (160cm)	=	9st 6lb (60kg)
5'4" (163cm)	=	7st 4lb (46.2kg)	5'4" (163cm)	=	8st 8lb (54.4kg)	5'4" (163cm)	=	9st 11lb (62.1kg)
5'5" (165cm)	=	7st 8lb (48kg)	5'5" (165cm)	=	8st 13lb (56.6kg)	5'5" (165cm)	=	10st 4lb (65.3kg)
5'6" (168cm)	=	7st 12lb (49.8kg)	5'6" (168cm)	=	9st 4lb (59kg)	5'6" (168cm)	=	10st 10lb (68kg)
5'7" (170cm)	=	8st 3lb (52kg)	5'7" (170cm)	=	9st 9lb (61kg)	5'7" (170cm)	=	11st 1lb (70kg)
5'8" (173cm)	=	8st 7lb (54kg)	5'8" (173cm)	=	10st (63.5kg)	5'8" (173cm)	=	11st 7lb (73kg)
5'9" (175cm)	=	8st 11lb (55.8kg)	5'9" (175cm)	=	10st 5lb (65.7kg)	5'9" (175cm)	=	11st 13lb (75.7kg)
5'10" (178cm)	=	9st 2lb (58kg)	5'10" (178cm)	=	10st 10lb (68kg)	5'10" (178cm)	=	12st 5lb (78.4kg)
5'11" (180cm)	=	9st 6lb (60kg)	5'11" (180cm)	=	11st 1lb (70kg)	5'11" (180cm)	=	12st 10lb (80.7kg)
6' (183cm)	=	9st 10lb (61.6kg)	6' (183cm)	=	11st 6lb (72.5kg)	6' (183cm)	=	13st 2lb (83.4kg)

Men

SMALL-BONED FRAME			MIDPOINT			LARGE-BONED FRAME		
5' (152cm)	=	6st 10lb (42.6kg)	5' (152cm)	=	7st 12lb (49.8kg)	5' (152cm)	=	9st 1lb (57.6kg)
5'1" (155cm)	=	7st 1lb (45kg)	5'1" (155cm)	=	8st 4lb (52.6kg)	5'1" (155cm)	=	9st 7lb (60kg)
5'2" (157cm)	=	7st 6lb (47kg)	5'2" (157cm)	=	8st 10lb (55.3kg)	5'2" (157cm)	=	10st (63.5kg)
5'3" (160cm)	=	7st 11lb (50kg)	5'3" (160cm)	=	9st 2lb (58kg)	5'3" (160cm)	=	10st 7lb (66.6kg)
5'4" (163cm)	=	8st 2lb (51.7kg)	5'4" (163cm)	=	9st 8lb (60.7kg)	5'4" (163cm)	=	11st (70kg)
5'5" (165cm)	=	8st 7lb (54kg)	5'5" (165cm)	=	10st (63.5kg)	5'5" (165cm)	=	11st 7lb (73kg)
5'6" (168cm)	=	8st 12lb (56kg)	5'6" (168cm)	=	10st 6lb (66kg)	5'6" (168cm)	=	12st (76kg)
5'7" (170cm)	=	9st 3lb (58.5kg)	5'7" (170cm)	=	10st 12lb (69kg)	5'7" (170cm)	=	12st 7lb (79.3kg)
5'8" (173cm)	=	9st 8lb (60.7kg)	5'8" (173cm)	=	11st 4lb (71.6kg)	5'8" (173cm)	=	13st (82.5kg)
5'9" (175cm)	=	9st 13lb (63kg)	5'9" (175cm)	=	11st 10lb (74kg)	5'9" (175cm)	=	13st 7lb (85.7kg)
5'10" (178cm)	=	10st 5lb (65.7kg)	5'10" (178cm)	=	12st 2lb (77kg)	5'10" (178cm)	=	14 (89kg)
5'11" (180cm)	=	10st 10lb (68kg)	5'11" (180cm)	=	12st 8lb (80kg)	5'11" (180cm)	=	14st 6lb (91.6kg)
6' (183cm)	=	11st 1lb (70kg)	6' (183cm)	=	13st (82.5kg)	6' (183cm)	=	14st 13lb (95kg)
6'1" (185cm)	=	11st 6lb (72.5kg)	6'1" (185cm)	=	13st 6lb (85kg)	6'1" (185cm)	=	15st 6lb (98kg)
6'2" (188cm)	=	11st 11lb (75kg)	6'2" (188cm)	=	13st 12lb (88kg)	6'2" (188cm)	=	15st 13lb (101kg)
6'3" (191cm)	=	12st 2lb (77kg)	6'3" (191cm)	=	14st 4lb (91kg)	6'3" (191cm)	=	16st 6lb (104kg)
6'4" (193cm)	=	12st 7lb (79.3kg)	6'4" (193cm)	=	14st 10lb (93kg)	6'4" (193cm)	=	16st 13lb (107.5kg)
6'5" (196cm)	=	12st 12lb (81.6kg)	6'5" (196cm)	=	15st 2lb (96kg)	6'5" (196cm)	=	17st 6lb (110.6kg)
6'6" (198cm)	=	13st 3lb (84kg)	6'6" (198cm)	=	15st 8lb (99kg)	6'6" (198cm)	=	17st 13lb (114kg)

We all want a healthy set point. Fortunately, I designed the 10x10 Program to deliberately change your set point through:

- Consistent strength-training exercise that increases muscle mass. Your muscle mass decreases by 1 percent each year after you turn 30. Unless you're building muscle, your metabolism will also decrease. (Muscle is much more metabolically active than fat, so the more muscle you have, the faster your metabolism will be.)
- Reduced calorie intake.
- Protein at each meal, even in some snacks.

Your Biochemistry: Food Is a Drug

Food is a drug. It is as powerful as the prescription medications this country is addicted to. It can make you feel either great or terrible. Think about the definition of *drug*: a substance that causes physiological changes in your body. Food has that same effect. In fact, it can produce physical responses far more complex than any pharmaceutical ever could.

When you eat sweets for example, you can get a true high, feeling as uplifted and energetic as if you took a hit of something, because it releases dopamine, serotonin, and norepinephrine into the brain. Some of our favorite antidepressants like Zoloft and Prozac have the same effect. Just as you come down from a drug, you crash from sugar when it leaves your system.

You've learned that you don't have to be stuck with your DNA, but you may be surprised to find out just how much food can either fix you or hurt you. On the positive side, food can nourish and heal us inside and out. I picked the foods for this plan that have the greatest pharmacological effect on you, so you will feel a difference fast.

Like a drug, the food you ingest has a powerful, immediate influence on your biochemistry. After your first day on the 10x10 Program, you will feel the effects of what you have eaten. Your body's response system to these new "food chemicals" will be the beginning of a new patterning. It's like taking an old, broken-down house and rebuilding it with new, improved fixtures from the foundation up.

Here's an example of how well your body functions when you eat something healthy, like a piece of fish. As soon as you put it in your mouth and chew, digestive enzymes start breaking down protein. The small intestines break down valuable amino acids that are carried by blood to the body's tissues. Not only do amino acids build protein (muscle) and collagen (beautiful skin), but some also increase serotonin, which makes you happy and peaceful. The more muscle you have, the better your body burns fat. So the digestion and absorption of protein are indirectly related to how well your body burns fat. And if the fish was salmon, a lot of the fat in it goes to the brain, to help manufacture neurotransmitters, brain chemicals. Your brain relies on about 50 different neurotransmitters. Examples include the following:

- Acetylcholine (ACh) affects brain activity related to attention, learning, and memory.
- Dopamine stimulates feelings of pleasure and affects arousal levels.
- Endorphins reduce stress and ease pain.
- Glutamate plays a vital role in learning and long-term memory.
- Noradrenaline stimulates mental and physical arousal and heightens mood.
- Serotonin affects mood levels, sleep, appetite, and other functions.

Scary Dairy

Why don't I have much dairy on my diet? We've been thoroughly conditioned to believe that milk is the perfect food. But it's not. You will never see me doing the "Got Milk" campaign because I am against having cow's milk as part of your diet (except a dash in coffee). We just don't need it in our diets. There's an overwhelming amount of research regarding cow's milk and how it damages our health. I know I'm treading on sacred ground here, but take a look at some of the facts I've found.

✓ Reactions to milk have been implicated in conditions including cirrhosis, asthma, eczema, arthritis, and irritable bowel syndrome. Dairy consumption has also been linked to heart disease, strokes, diabetes, and obesity.

✓ The bodies of around 75 percent of the world's population lack the correct enzyme to digest milk, so when it makes its way into their digestive systems it wreaks havoc, causing digestive distress, inflammation, bloating, and other problems.

✓ There have been suggestions that milk drinkers may have an increased risk of breast cancer from the bovine growth hormones (BGH) given to dairy cows.

✓ Ovarian cancer, a particularly difficult cancer to diagnose and treat, has been associated with dairy products. Milk drinkers appear to have a 3.1 percent greater risk than non–milk drinkers.

Continued

✓ Rather than stopping osteoporosis, milk actually encourages it, says a Harvard study. It followed some 75,000 nurses and found that the more milk they drank, the greater chance they had of developing brittle bone disease. Milk is loaded with acid proteins, which leach calcium away from the bones. You want calcium? Get it from veggies like greens, cabbage, ocean vegetables, chickpeas, red beans, and broccoli.

Love milk? Fine, but instead of cow's milk, try almond or rice milk. Both taste great and can be substituted practically anywhere for cow's milk.

The most important stop is the liver, because it is the organ most responsible for metabolizing fat. The liver can also pump excess fat out of the body through the bile into the small intestines. If your diet is high in fiber, this unwanted fat will be carried out of the body via the bowel actions. Thus, the liver is a remarkable machine for keeping weight under control, being both a fat-burning and a fat-flushing organ.

So you see, food is broken down into tiny molecules that control your body and brain. That's exactly what drugs do. You need to start thinking of foods as either bad drugs or good drugs. Vegetables, whole grains, and fish are among the good drugs.

Processed or fake foods are bad drugs. I'm talking about additives and chemicals. Did you know artificial ingredients can actually make you fat even if they have no fat or calories in them? When you eat or drink something, your body processes it appropriately by using what it needs and getting rid of the rest. But our bodies weren't designed to process chemicals and other artificial ingredients. When you ingest one, the body doesn't know exactly what to do with it. So what it does is surround that mystery mass in fat and tuck it away someplace you'd probably rather it not be, like your belly.

Okay, so now you see the power of food to change your chemistry, make you happier, and stop disease in its tracks. **Your fridge is like a pharmacy. Make healthy food your drug of choice.**

Sleep Cycles and Weight Loss

Insomnia and stress are two conditions that will halt your weight loss in a heartbeat. While you sleep, your body restores itself from all of the stressors and junk you've put into it emotionally and physically during the day. All the women in my family suffer from terrible insomnia. I have spent my life trying to solve this issue.

You may think you are getting proper sleep, but there is a deep REM state that many of us do not get enough of. That lack can leave us tired and make us gain weight. Our pituitary glands crank out the highest levels of growth hormones while we are in deep sleep. Growth hormone is a multitasker. It repairs damaged tissues, burns fat, and builds muscle. It is known as the youth hormone; people spend millions in rejuvenation therapies like human growth hormone (HGH) injections in an effort to supplement it. If we don't sleep well, the stimulating hormones adrenaline and noradrenaline are triggered. They wipe out the benefits of growth hormone. No amount of daytime sleep will make up for the nighttime sleep loss, because the energy needed for tissue repair is not available during daylight hours—it's being used elsewhere in the body.

If you wake up at 4 AM or so every night, that is usually an indication of an abnormal cortisol spike. Cortisol is a stress hormone most associated

Don't Sleep, Get Fat

According to Columbia University's New York Obesity Research Center, women who slept only four hours a night ate an average of 329 calories more the following day than when they were well rested. For men, it was 263 calories. If these extra calories were consumed daily, it would equal a yearly weight gain of about 2st 5lb (15kg) for the women and 1st 13lb (12kg) pounds for the men.

with belly fat, a hot topic plastered on the covers of most health and fitness magazines. Cortisol spikes occur with unresolved stress and imbalance in the body from—you guessed it—improper diet and no exercise. By eating five times throughout the day, including breakfast, you'll lower cortisol production and decrease the chance you'll overeat throughout the day.

My 10x10 plan focuses on whole foods. These are unprocessed foods (like whole-grain bread and fresh vegetables) and are the least likely to stimulate cortisol. Whole foods contain fiber and nutrients that help keep your blood sugar levels steady; they are the mainstay of my diet.

Sleep problems also affect the balance of two hunger-related hormones: leptin, which is released by fat cells, signaling the brain to *stop* eating, and ghrelin (pronounced *GRELL-in*), which is made in the stomach and tells the brain to *keep* eating. Both hormones influence whether you go for a second helping or push yourself away from the table. Lots of research shows that leptin levels are lower and ghrelin levels are higher in people who who don't sleep an adequate number of hours.

So rest easy tonight and know that my 10x10 Program is designed to help resolve your sleep issues.

Your Thinking: Get Headstrong

Do you want a quick fix or do you want a lasting change for a lifetime? The only way to lose weight and keep it off is by addressing the whole person.

Here's a question I ask my clients: What do you think you have to do to succeed on this program? I usually hear answers like: Stop eating so much, sacrifice my wine nights, stop eating desserts. Some even say "Be disciplined," or "Punish myself with hard workouts." There is a whole lot of talk about deprivation and punishment; a life pursuing wellness sounds more like a walk to the gallows than achieving peace and happiness.

This kind of negative thinking sets you up to fail. If exercise and sticking to a healthy diet are perceived as drudgery, no matter how many times you try to force yourself into sticking to your plan, in the end you'll find ways to go back to the things that make you feel good in the moment but very bad in the long run. When you feel angry about having to feel a burn or eat healthy foods, you will find ways to sabotage yourself. It's so important that you start now to link all good things with the

Develop Muscle, Improve Body Image

Researchers with the *Journal of Applied Sport Psychology* put a group of women on a 13-week weight-training program and compared them with a group not working out. The weight trainers displayed body-image improvements, felt better about themselves, and no longer were classified as body-image-disturbed.

program and all negative thoughts with not working the program. A beautiful, strong body will follow; after that come more confidence, better connections with people, and doors of opportunity flying open for you. Look at every change I'm asking you to embrace as a gift, not a chore. Making the decision to get into the best shape of your life should be exciting and energizing.

Now that I've told you a bit about the 10x10 Diet, let me fill you in on the details of the fitness program and how it helps you take off 10lb (4.5kg) in ten days, too.

CHAPTER 3

The 10x10 Fitness Program

Gearing Up to Work Out

HOW YOU HANDLE A WORKOUT SESSION is very similar to how you should handle your life. As in life, you need to set a goal (rep or set) and see it through to the end. You know there will be some pain, but you push through because the result is growth (muscle tone). And the hard work always pays off with a reward (body change).

Believe You Can Do It

The first step to achieving that is believing that you can do these workouts. Never say "I'll try"—just *do*! I don't let any of my clients get away with passive or noncommittal talk in the gym. Your workouts will connect you to your body even more than sex does. It is your time to envision your body as the beautiful machine that it is. Instead of focusing on being fat, focus on being fit. If you think healthy, it eventually becomes reality for you. There is nothing sexier than feeling strong and carrying yourself with strength.

Stay Focused on Results

Focus on how strong you're getting, how well you're sleeping, and how happy you're feeling. Choosing to focus on thoughts that feel good, and are positive, is a sure way to create the body you want. The by-product is beauty. Do not "hope to," but assume you *will* lose weight. Great things come to those who work for a goal and assume the outcome will be in their favor. You'll be sending out the right energy, and it's energy that creates your new reality. **Change your mind and your body will follow.**

My custom-designed weight-training and cardio routines are challenging, and they advance as you do. There comes a point in your training when your growth is basically going to stop unless you're really changing up the components of your program. Here, you'll be constantly challenged to burn fat and calories, tone and strengthen. After all, your goal is not only to lose 10lb (4.5kg) over the next ten days, but also to find your strength. My workout program will get you there.

Thrive on More Energy

Exercise is energy-giving. You won't want to sit on your butt when you feel so instantly great after your workouts. My workouts are so kick-ass and effective that your body has no choice but to get lean and beautiful. I pulled the exercises and combos right from my personal training log, and you've seen what they've done for me. The workouts I've designed are plateau-busting routines that force your body to continuously burn fat while putting on lean muscle. You'll do this primarily through resistance training and cardio bursts. The only way to change your genetic shape is through resistance training. You're about to learn to train exactly like I do!

Now, if you've seen me train people in the past, you know two things: You'll need to give an all-out intense effort and push beyond your perceived physical limits, and because of that, you'll get real, inspirational results. **My goal is to get you excited about learning new styles of training so you can confidently walk into any gym and feel strong.**

Exercise Is a Drug, Too

Remember what I said about food being a drug? Well, exercise is a drug, too. Exercise literally changes brain biochemistry. The blood and energy supply to your brain improves. The genes in nerve cells signal the production of special proteins that induce nerve cells to grow, branch, and make connections with one another. It's a process called neuroplasticity. I bet you bought into the myth that once you lose brain cells, they're gone for good. Well, exercise brings them back in a process called neurogenesis.

Exercise is an amazing, natural antidepressant. Going back to genetics, if either of your parents or any grandparents suffered from depression, anxiety, or mood instability, you are prone to suffer as well. Depression runs in my family, and I suffered greatly until I changed my lifestyle. I have been living drug-free ever since, and when I miss my workout for two to three days the blues start creeping in. Exercise can literally save your life! It makes you feel good, think better, and feel emotionally stronger.

Right after you start exercising, the brain invigorates certain chemicals that reinforce pleasure, boost mood, and help you overcome fear and anxiety. For instance:

- *Serotonin* boosts your mood.
- *Dopamine* is a pleasure-producing chemical. (Yes, exercise is pleasure boosting, thanks to this chemical!)

- *Epinephrine* and *norepinephrine* are two hormones released quickly after exercise that put immune cells on active alert, accelerating their response to an invasion from germs.
- *Endogenous opioids* are narcotic-like substances produced by the body and are known to be involved in the reduction of fear.

You should understand by now that with the powerful combo of food and exercise, at any age you can build a better brain, which works for you instead of against you!

Should Women Train Like Men?

Now, women, I know what you're thinking: *I don't want to lift heavy weights and end up looking like a man.* Here's the truth: Your body is predisposed to put on muscle a certain way in certain places, just like it puts on fat. You will never look like a man because you don't have anywhere close to the amount of testosterone men have. Testosterone, coupled with heavy weights, results in increased muscle size and the typical "manly" physique. There are places in all of us that build quicker than others. That is why it's so important to have a balanced routine that focuses on all muscle groups evenly. Ask yourself this question: *Do I want to have a firm and shapely body under those jeans, or a loose, flabby body?*

You need to put those worries aside and trust that I designed the 10x10 Fitness Program with toning and fat burning in mind, not power lifting. You are training to be stronger, healthier, better looking, more youthful, and more proficient in daily activities. My style of training makes that happen. I feel that in terms of program design and intensity, women and men should train identically. If you train like a man, you'll reach your goals faster.

Use Your Shape to Your Advantage

If you train and eat exactly like me, can you expect to develop an identical physique? Not unless you are my genetic body type, which is tall, lanky, and resistant to putting on muscle weight. I have to kill it in the gym every day in order to get this body because I am an ectomorph, and ectomorphs have a hard time building muscle.

We all come in different sizes and shapes. You have a genetically predetermined body type as ectomorph, endomorph, mesomorph, or, more likely, some combination thereof. You can find out which one you are by taking a good, hard look in the mirror.

ECTOMORPH: This is me! I call it the "scrawny man or woman." You are typically skinny and find it very hard to put on muscle. Ectos have a slight build with small joints. Usually ectomorphs have long, thin limbs with stringy muscles. Shoulders tend to be thin with little width.

ENDOMORPH: You gain fat very easily and are generally soft and round. You have a stockier appearance and tend to look more apple-shaped. It is harder to lose fat but your muscles are strong, especially in the upper legs.

MESOMORPH: You have a large bone structure, large muscles, and a naturally athletic physique. Most of the fitness competitors you see have this body type, which is the best type for bodybuilding. They find it quite easy to gain and lose weight. Women are hourglass-shaped, and men tend to look rectangular.

Stop focusing on having a completely different body and focus on having the best body that is yours. Your body type is pretty much determined on the day you are born. You can't change your bone structure, but you can change your shape with resistance training. What is distinctive about the 10x10 Fitness Program is that it works for all body types. You get the exact right kind of cardio and strength training that burns fat and gives you the best shape for your body type.

How Exercise Burns Fat

There are a lot of ways the body burns fat—too much physiology to cover here. But I do want to give you a brief glimpse into how exercise burns fat—and can even burn fat in specific areas of the body.

You may have heard that you can't spot-reduce, only spot-tone, but we now know that both can occur. Basically, when fat is burned by exercise, blood picks up fat and carries it to exercising muscle fibers to be burned for fuel. An increase in blood flow to fat cells means that more fat has been removed from fat cells and delivered to muscles for use as fuel during exercise. Using high repetitions with little rest in between will give you the best toning-and-reduction combo to change your genetic shape.

Intensity Techniques

I know you're ready to commit yourself to the 10x10 Fitness Program. Just thinking about the changes you're going to make in strength, size, endurance, and general health should start that inner fire and motivate you. As you read and learn more about my training techniques, you'll come across terminology that is key to your continued progress. The more you understand these variables and how to manipulate them in your workouts, the more steadily you'll progress toward your goals without experiencing the usual plateaus.

I started getting into weight training at about 21 years old. I began by reading *Muscle and Fitness* magazine. I didn't understand the science and terminology of exercise, but I quickly learned that if I tore out the exercises and did them as many times and as many days as I read that I should, I would feel sore and I would reshape my body (I was a scrawny weakling). The more excited and immersed in the culture of fitness I got, the more I tried to understand about exercise. As you can see,

On the Spot

New research from the University of Copenhagen suggests that spot reduction can really happen. Danish researchers had ten male subjects perform one-leg extensions for 30 minutes with a fairly light weight. Blood flow was jacked up in the fat cells of the exercising leg compared with the resting leg. So basically, the body was burning thigh fat as a result of exercise.

there's a lot more to training than you probably thought. But that's what's so exciting about my 10x10 Fitness Program—you can manipulate so many things in your workouts, they'll never get boring. As you start my program, you're more than likely going to make progress right away. That's because you're doing something new and your body is eager to adapt to this new activity.

Here are the fat-burning workout principles that you need to know, and they further explain why this exercise program works so powerfully. When you put these exercise tricks to work, you will turn on your inner athlete and fully commit to your body.

Intensity Technique 1
Cardio-Acceleration

Cardio-acceleration is a short but intense cardio burst inbetween your strength-training exercises. It is one of the quickest ways to burn fat in a routine that combines strength training and aerobics.

I'm building your cardio right into your resistance-training sessions by having you skipping rope between specified exercises. It works like this: Between exercise sets, you'll do either 100 or 200 rotations depending on what program you are on. These fat-burning bursts of exercise will make a big difference in your results.

Cardio-Acceleration Is a Proven Fat Burner

Researchers at the University of California at Berkeley and Santa Cruz studied two different types of workouts. The first was one hour of traditional strength training followed by 30 minutes of cardiovascular exercise. The second was a combined strength-and-cardio workout (cardio-acceleration). The second group of exercisers saw an almost tenfold greater reduction in body fat compared with the first group, and also saw an 82.2 percent increase in muscle gain.

Intensity Technique 2
HIIT
(High-Intensity Interval Training)

The mistake a lot of people make is doing too much cardio, and the wrong kind, such as one-hour-plus treadmill runs. The most effective and time-efficient cardio is interval cardio: alternating bursts of high-intensity and lower-intensity aerobic activity. While the intensity burns up lots of calories, the recovery periods inbetween draw energy straight from your fat stores, providing a two-pronged effect.

You'll do interval cardio twice in ten days, on a day you don't weight train.

Intensity Technique 3
Supersets

When I train my clients, I like to be quick and efficient. I want to challenge their cardiovascular and neuromuscular systems simultaneously, and I want them to work not only hard but also smart. That's why I believe that supersets are a fantastic training principle. With this technique, you do sets of two different exercises for the same muscle group back-to-back, then two more exercises for a different muscle group, taking no rest between. So a superset is like one long extended set, only it consists of four different movements. This fast training will help rev your metabolism and trigger fat loss.

Intensity Technique 4
Full-Body Circuit

Twice during each ten-day period, you'll perform full-body circuit training—doing ten or more exercises virtually nonstop, going from one exercise to the next and alternating muscle groups. This style of circuit training increases lean mass and aerobic capacity while reducing body fat. The continuous nature of circuit training keeps your metabolism high throughout the workout.

Also, when you train using a circuit, your cardiovascular system can be strengthened. Your heart, also a muscle, pumps blood more efficiently. The smooth muscles around arteries and veins become more elastic. This fights hardening of the arteries and helps lower blood pressure.

Intensity Technique 5
Rest-Pause to 100 Reps

This method involves stopping when you've reached failure in a set, resting for a short period of time, then continuing for as many reps as you can before failing again. Continue until you reach 100 reps total.

Forced Reps Force Fat Burning

Finnish researchers studied 16 male athletes after one of two leg workouts. The standard workout consisted of 12 reps to failure. The forced-rep workout used heavier weight and needed a spotter to complete 12 reps. The forced-rep program produced much higher GH levels. This means that, hormonally, forced reps shift your body into a fat-burning mode.

Six-Pack Abs

You'll notice throughout the ten days that the abdominal movements come at the end of your workouts. It is important to not weaken your core too much before strengthening your other muscle groups, because your core musculature maintains spinal alignment. If you train your abs first and fatigue them, it hinders your body's ability to protect the spine and puts you at risk for injury. I'm known to say, "Crunches are a waste of time." Now, I don't mean that ab work should be ignored. A strong core is the key to strong limbs. Squats and push-ups are actually a much better way to lose abdominal fat, because the chest and legs are primary muscle groups and are larger. Remember, the more muscle you have on your frame, the more fat you will burn even as you sleep, so it makes sense to focus on those fat-burning muscles. Doing 300 crunches without focusing on primary muscles will just build under that layer of belly fat, and you may even look bigger.

Progress and Plateaus

Hey, we've all had times when our progress came to a screeching halt and we were just going through the motions during our workouts. Don't sweat it, because the chance of plateaus on the 10x10 Fitness Program is zero.

Why? Because there's so much variety built into the training routines. In the past, you might have hit plateaus because you did the same old thing too many times. You may not fully realize this, but your body adapts very quickly to the demands you place upon it. Add more weight to your exercises and your body quickly adapts by growing firmer and

Plateau Busters

Plateau Buster 1: Overload

Overload is the amount of stress you put on a muscle. The body is amazing at adapting to stress. When you start your resistance-training program, the body will change in ways that leave it better able to handle that stress the next time it occurs. So if you want your muscles to grow, for example, you must increase the stress you put on them by increasing your weights.

Plateau Buster 2: Volume

This refers to the amount of work you do, like the number of sets and reps. You can increase volume in several ways:

- Keep the reps the same, but increase the number of sets.
- Keep the sets the same, but change the number of reps per set.
- Count the total number of sets and reps you do in a workout, a week, or a month, and make adjustments from there.

As you advance, have fun with these manipulations—they keep your training motivation high, and you'll be able to see how each change affects your body.

stronger muscles. Reduce the rest time between sets and your body quickly adapts by making you more cardiovascularly fit. The way to overcome this adaptability is by constantly changing the way you train. You'll be changing your routine constantly with different exercise groupings and rep work that will continuously force change. Your body plateaus with resistance training and cardio in about one month, so you must change what you do frequently.

Plateau Buster 3: Intensity

How hard you train makes up the intensity of your workouts. Weight-lifting intensity is measured by how much you are lifting with good form to max repetitions. If you squat with 100lb (45kg) for five reps and then with 125lb (56kg) for five reps, the latter set is more intense than the former. And if you were to rest for two minutes between sets, the workout would be less intense than if you rested one minute between sets. Intensity applies to aerobic exercise, too. The more elevated your heart rate, the higher your intensity.

Plateau Buster 4: Frequency

Here I'm talking about how often you train—more specifically, how often you do a particular exercise or train a certain body part. Frequency can be measured in terms of each training day, week, or even an entire month. When you follow a program, one of the things you can manipulate is how many times a week you want to go to the gym and how often you want to train each body part. My program has weight training with frequency—six days a week. The more often you train, the more fat you burn.

Plateau Buster 5: Duration

Change:

- How long it takes you to complete the allotted number of sets for an exercise
- How long a particular training session lasts
- How long it takes you to train a body part
- The length of an entire training program

Apply these plateau busters for a lifetime and you will be fit for a lifetime!

Understanding How to Read the 10x10 Fitness Program

Simple Equipment to Get Started!

I always keep my workouts super-simple, so you need only two pieces of equipment for this program: a skipping rope and dumbbells. You can purchase these items anywhere sporting goods are sold.

Skipping Rope

Minute for minute, using a skipping rope is one of the most beneficial exercises a person can participate in. It is an unparalleled cardiovascular workout that will tone and strengthen your entire body. Here are a few ways to get the most out of your rope:

- Keep your arm position relaxed, and try to make small circles. Keep the arms close to your torso, turning your forearms and wrists in a cranking motion.
- Jump only a few inches off the ground, leaving just enough room to let the rope pass under your feet. *Remember that skipping is about timing, not how high you jump.* Jumping too high off the ground causes you to use a lot of excess energy and to land with way too much impact. You're pushing up off the balls of your feet; your heels are just tapping the ground.
- Turn the rope fast enough to jump a full revolution. Try not to add an extra bunny hop between revolutions because you are going too slow.

Dumbbells

Suggested Starting Weight

Biceps/Triceps/Shoulders:

Women—A pair of 6lb or 8lb (2.7kg or 3.6kg) dumbbells

Men—A pair of 15lb or 20lb (6.7kg or 9kg) dumbbells

Legs/Chest/Back:

Women—A pair of 12lb or 15lb (5.4kg or 6.7kg) dumbbells

Men—A pair of 25lb or 35lb (11.2kg or 15.8kg) dumbbells

If you can perform ten reps without a pretty intense burn on the last three to five, then you need to increase the weight you're using.

Workout Lingo

If you're going to do my program, you've got to be familiar with workout language. A quick read-through of the following terms, and you'll be fluent.

Rep: One complete motion of an exercise from starting position back to starting position.

Set: The specific number of reps you perform of one exercise.

Form: The correct technique involved in performing an exercise. This typically involves proper posture and control of reps. A mistake many exercisers make is performing reps with rapid, jerky movements. This adds no real resistance and can actually damage your joints. *Slow it down!*

Routine: The complete series of exercises that you perform during your workout. A whole-body routine can be done in one session and repeated several times per week. Other routines are "split routines," in which you work certain body parts like chest and triceps in one workout; legs and abs in another; and back, biceps, and shoulders in a third, with each body-part workout done on a different day.

Rest Periods

One of the common mistakes I see in the gym is that people rest too long between exercises. The whole point of circuit training for optimal fat loss is that you keep your heart rate up.

During Phase 1 of your 10x10 supersets, try to take only 10 or 15 seconds of rest between the movements; after completing all four, go ahead and take a longer rest of about 30 to 45 seconds before and after using your skipping rope. Resting 30 seconds between sets has been shown to increase caloric burn by 50 percent, compared with a three-minute rest period. So put yourself through the paces; the added calorie burn is worth it.

Split Routines

If you've usually trained all your muscle groups in a single workout session, now you'll split up your routine so you work different body parts on different days, giving some muscles much-needed rest while working others.

For example, on the first-day split you'll train your chest, biceps, and abs; on the second-day split, your shoulders, legs, and abs; and on the third-day split, your back, triceps, and abs.

Split routines let your body recover better, which results in more tone and more fat burning throughout the day.

Finding Your Inner Athlete

What Is Confidence?

Confidence is your belief in your ability to succeed. Work on creating mental strength strategies to build confidence by looking for success. Success can come from achieving a training goal you set for yourself or going for your morning run when you really want to stay in bed. Just setting a goal of drinking two to three liters of water a day and achieving that goal create success.

Another effective means of developing confidence is through the process of modeling, or copying the success of others; what one can do, any can do. This is why I constantly refer to what works for me: so you can copy what I do and achieve the wellness and balance I've now attained.

I have said for years, "Fake it till you make it." I have done this to combat my natural shyness, and it got me jobs that I was not the most qualified for.

Your thoughts, feelings, and behaviors are always linked. If you act confident, this will help trigger a confident mind-set. A simple way to fake confidence is to practice how you walk into a room. Always make eye contact with others and smile. Always walk "tall," with your chest out, shoulders back with authority. Your energy will cut through like a knife in any space that you occupy.

Every time you have failure thoughts, redirect to positive. If you hear that inner saboteur saying *I can't do this workout*, for instance, tell yourself, *This workout is going to make me strong and fit*. See how that works? Apply that thinking to everything and you will start being your biggest champion.

The Exercises

I have chosen five warm-up exercises, 30 different weight-lifting exercises, and five cool-down movements. I want you to master these basic movements in a short amount of time so that you can move from one superset to another by memory. They are organized by muscle group.

The Warm-Up Routine

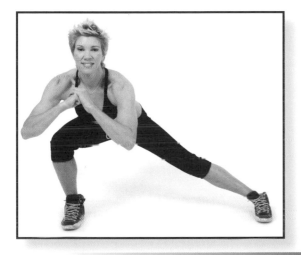 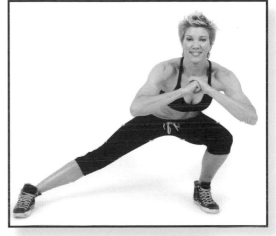

Side-to-Side Lunge

- Stand with your feet wide, toes out at about a 45-degree angle.
- Lunge to the right, bending your knee and taking care to keep the knee behind the toe.
- Repeat the lunge on the left side. Do 10 reps. One rep is a lunge to the right and left.

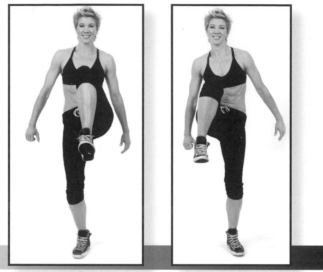

Knee-Up

- Lift your left knee up to chest level. Lower.
- Then lift your right knee up to chest level.
- Alternate like this for 10 reps on each knee. Keep your abs engaged as you perform the warm-up.

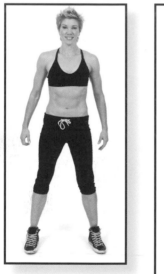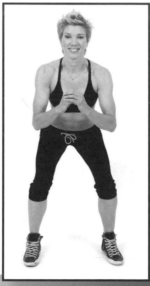

Leg Warm-Up

- Stand with your legs about shoulder-width apart and your hands at your sides.
- Flex your knees and squat slightly as you bring your hands up and together in front of your chest.
- Continue for 10 repetitions.

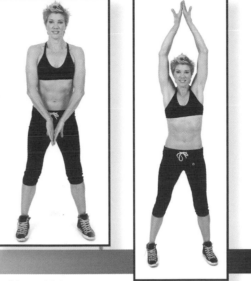

Shoulder Warm-Up

- Stand with your feet about shoulder-width apart, with your hands in front of you, palms inverted outward.
- Raise your arms overhead, as shown, stretching your torso as you go.
- Continue for 10 repetitions.

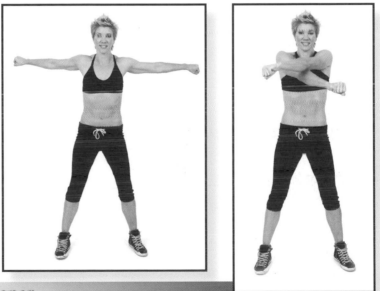

Chest Opener

- Stand with your feet about shoulder-width apart and your arms outstretched to your sides.
- Rapidly cross straight arms in front of you.
- Continue for 10 repetitions.

Chest Exercises

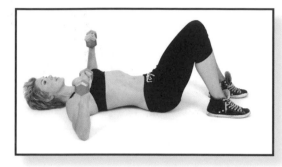 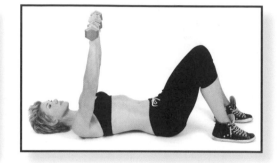

Flat Press

- Lie faceup on your back.
- Place your feet flat on the floor.
- Hold a dumbbell in each hand in a neutral position.
- Slowly bend your elbows to a 90-degree angle until the dumbbells are just above your chest.
- Lift the dumbbells until your arms are extended above your midchest.
- Slowly lower the dumbbells in a straight line down to your chest.
- Press back up and repeat the motion.

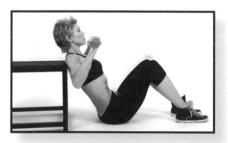 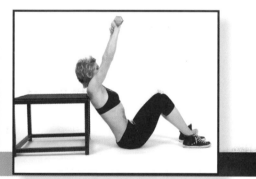

Incline Press

- Lean back against a couch or bench at an angle of roughly 30 to 45 degrees.
- Angle your body face-forward with your feet flat on the floor.
- Hold a dumbbell in each hand just outside your shoulders.
- Powerfully press the dumbbells upward toward the ceiling, stopping when the dumbbells are 1 inch (2cm) away from each other.
- Slowly return the dumbbells to the starting position and repeat.

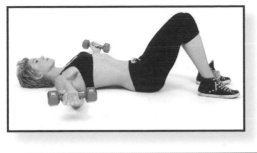
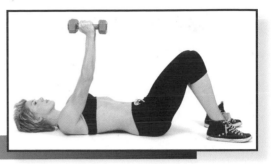

Flat Flye

- Hold a dumbbell in each hand and lie on your back.
- With your palms facing each other, extend your arms straight up so that the dumbbells are directly over your chest.
- Slightly bend your elbows and extend them downward in an arc until you feel a complete stretch in your upper chest.
- Hold the open position for a pause.
- Now squeeze your chest muscles and draw your arms back to the starting position.

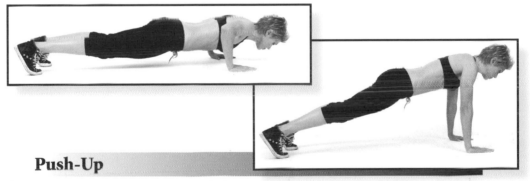

Push-Up

- Place the palms of your hands flat on the floor at shoulder level and slightly more than shoulder-width apart.
- Place your feet together and parallel to each other.
- Keep your legs and body straight and your toes tucked under your feet.
- Slowly lower your body until your chest is 3–4 inches (7–10cm) from the ground.
- Pause and push yourself up.

Back Exercises

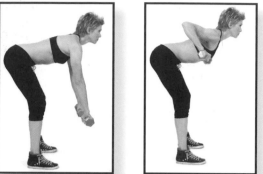

Bent-Over Wide Row

- Lean forward so that your torso is at about a 90-degree angle to the floor. Keep your knees slightly bent.
- Hold a dumbbell in each hand, palms toward your body, with arms straight. Raise the dumbbells by pulling your arms up and toward your spine, bringing your elbows as high as you can. Squeeze your back muscles briefly at the top of the pull.
- Lower the weight along the same path.

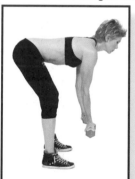 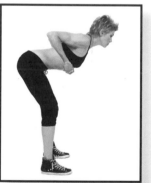

Reverse-Grip Row

- Lean forward so that your torso is at about a 90-degree angle to the floor. Keep your knees slightly bent.
- Hold a dumbbell in each hand with a reverse grip so that your palms are facing forward and your arms are straight.
- Slowly pull the weights up toward your chest until you cannot contract the muscles any further and your shoulder blades are squeezed together.
- Return to the starting position.

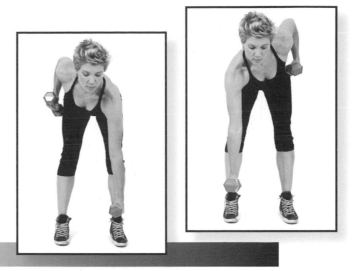

Alternating Row

- Lean forward so that your torso is at about a 90-degree angle to the floor.
- Hold a dumbbell in each hand, palms facing each other, arms straight. Raise the right dumbbell by pulling your arm up and toward your spine, bringing your elbow as high as you can. Squeeze your back muscles briefly at the top, then lower the weight along the same path.
- Repeat with your left arm. Alternate right and left arms until the rep set is complete.

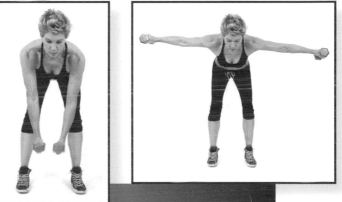

Rear Lateral Raise

- Lean forward so that your torso is at about a 90-degree angle to the floor with your feet shoulder-width apart.
- Grasp a dumbbell in each hand, holding them with your palms facing each other.
- Bend your elbows slightly, and raise the dumbbells up and outward until they are slightly higher than shoulder height.
- Return to the starting position.

Leg Exercises

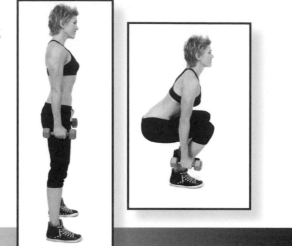

Deep Squat

- Stand with your feet a little wider than shoulder-width apart and your knees slightly bent.
- Hold a dumbbell in each hand for increased resistance.
- Keeping your head neutral, abs tight, and torso erect, bend at the knees and hips to slowly lower your body as if you were going to sit down in a chair. Your thighs should be parallel to the floor.
- Straighten your legs to the starting position, pressing back up from your heels.

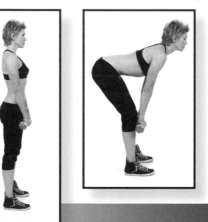

Deadlift

- Stand with your feet shoulder-width apart and a dumbbell outside each leg.
- Keeping your knees slightly bent, lower the dumbbells in front of you just below your knees.
- Extend at the knees and hips to pull the dumbbells upward until you're at a standing position.
- Squeeze your back, legs, and glutes and repeat.

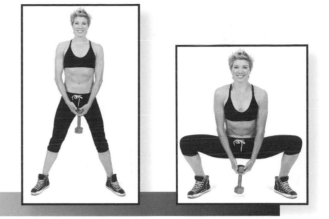

Sumo Squat

- Holding one dumbbell with both hands, stand with your feet wider apart than shoulder-width. Turn your toes out to 45 degrees. Keep your shoulders back and your hips tucked in.
- Slowly bend at the knees and lower your body until your hamstrings are parallel to the floor.
- Pause for a second in the bottom position; then push up through your heels to drive back up to the starting position.

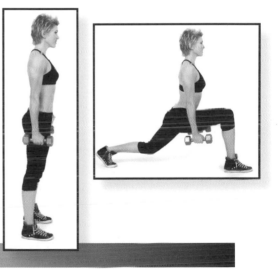

Front Alternating Lunge

- Begin with your feet together, your chest out, and your shoulders back. Hold a dumbbell in each hand at your sides.
- Take a big step forward on your right foot and lower the opposite knee to the ground.
- Push back to the starting position without bouncing. Make sure you put your weight on the lunging heel, not on your toe.
- Alternate to your left side, repeating the movement.

Arm Exercises: Biceps

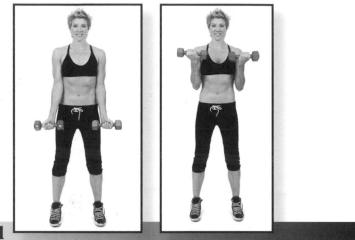

Biceps Curl

- Stand holding a dumbbell in each hand, palms forward.
- Keeping your chest up, curl both dumbbells up toward your shoulders.
- Squeeze your biceps hard at the top; then lower to the starting position.
- Repeat.

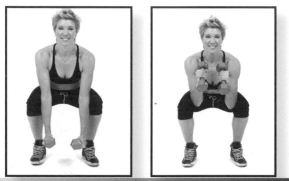

Close Hammer Curl

- Grasp a dumbbell in each hand.
- Stand with your arms hanging at your sides, palms facing inward.
- Bend your knees and squat down, as shown.
- Keep your arms close to your sides.
- Curl the dumbbells as high as you can go.
- Squeeze your biceps hard at the top of the lift. The top of the dumbbells should be pointing toward the ceiling.
- Lower the dumbbells to the resting position.

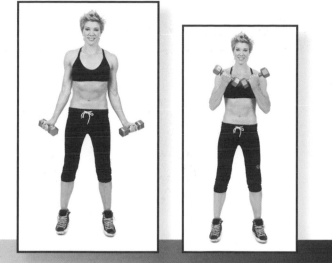

Diagonal Curl

- Stand holding the dumbbells in your hands with your palms facing forward.
- Place your feet slightly wider than your shoulders with your knees slightly bent.
- Raise your arms at the elbow, simultaneously turning your arm inward in a diagonal motion. The dumbbells should meet at the center of your chest.
- Slowly lower to the starting position.

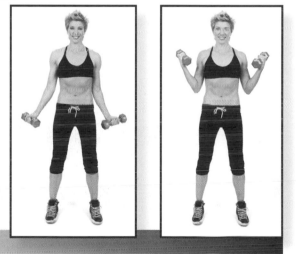

Outer Curl

- From a standing position, grasp a dumbbell in each hand, palms facing out to the sides.
- Keeping your upper arms close to your sides, curl the weights upward until you can't bend further.
- Squeeze your muscles at the top of the contraction.
- Lower slowly and repeat the movement.

Arm Exercises: Triceps

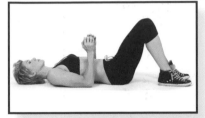 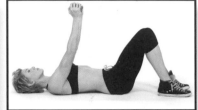

Close-Grip Press

- Lie on your back on the floor and grasp one dumbbell with both hands, with your palms facing each other.
- Straighten your arms and line them up directly above your lower chest. This is the starting position.
- Slowly lower the dumbbell until it touches your lower rib cage.
- Without pausing or bouncing at the bottom of the movement, push the dumbbell upward to full arm extension.

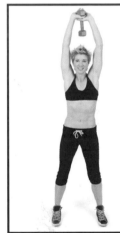 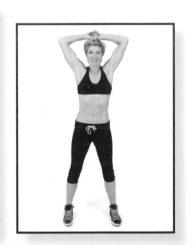

Single Headbanger

- Stand with your feet shoulder-width apart and grasp one dumbbell in both hands with an overhand grip.
- Hold the dumbbell with straight arms over and slightly behind the top of your head.
- Bend your elbows to lower the dumbbell until your forearms are just past parallel with the floor.
- Go back to straightened position.

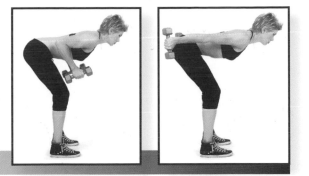

Kickback

- Bend over at the waist at a 90-degree angle.
- Holding a dumbbell in each hand, raise your upper arms to parallel your torso, keeping them pressed into your sides.
- Holding your upper arm in place, kick your lower arm straight back to full extension.
- Don't allow your elbow to drop as you return your lower arm to the starting position.

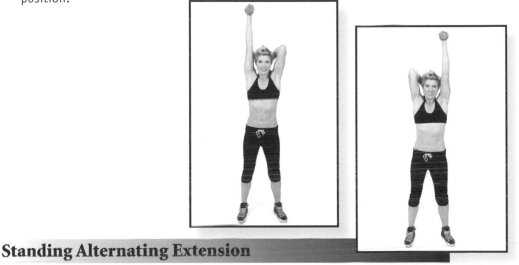

Standing Alternating Extension

- Grasp a dumbbell in each hand.
- Start with the dumbbells overhead.
- One at a time, lower the weight behind your head as deep as you can without letting it touch your upper back on the way down.
- Keep the upper part of your arm as close to your head and as vertical as possible throughout the movement.
- Repeat with the other arm, alternating each time.
- Keep the weight constantly moving; avoid resting in a lockout to keep constant tension on your triceps.

Shoulder Exercises

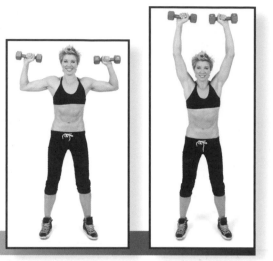

Military Press

- Stand holding a dumbbell in each hand at shoulder height, with your palms facing forward and your elbows directly under your hands.
- Keeping your back straight, press the dumbbells upward and slightly toward the midline of your body. Do not lock your elbows.
- Hold for a one-count at the top; then slowly lower the dumbbells to shoulder height.

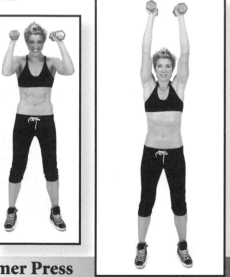

Hammer Press

- Hold the dumbbells in front of your head, elbows bent at 90 degrees and knuckles to the side.
- Press the weights above your head until your arms are straight.
- Lower to the starting position.

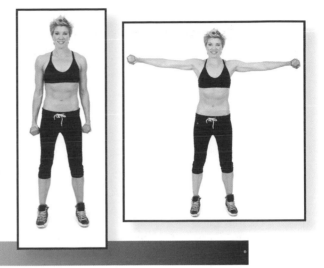

Lateral Raise

- Stand with your feet shoulder-width apart. Keep your abs tight, chest up, and shoulders back.
- Hold the dumbbells at your sides with your palms facing each other.
- Bend your elbows slightly. Raise the dumbbells up and outward until they are slightly higher than shoulder height. Hold momentarily.
- Slowly return to the starting position.

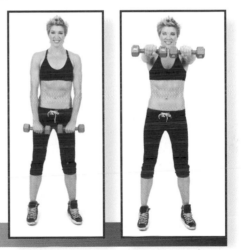

Front Raise

- Stand with your feet about shoulder-width apart.
- Grasp a dumbbell in each hand and hold them across your thighs. Do not lean back as you raise the weights.
- Lift the weights upward to your shoulder line, palms facing down, with your arms parallel to the floor.

Ab Exercises

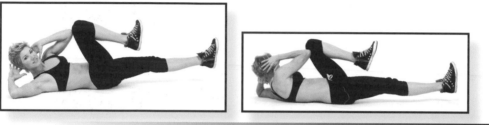

Bicycle

- Lie face up with your fingertips behind your head for light support.
- Bend your knees, with your feet flat on the floor or exercise mat.
- Simultaneously extend right leg and cross your right shoulder toward your left knee while pulling that knee in toward your chest.
- Touch your elbow to your knee.
- Alternate from side to side. Once to each side equals one rep.

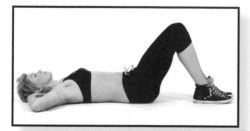
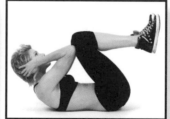

Reverse Crunch

- Lie on the floor with your hips and legs bent.
- With your hands behind your head, come up in a crunching motion until your knees and elbows make contact.
- Slowly return to the starting position.

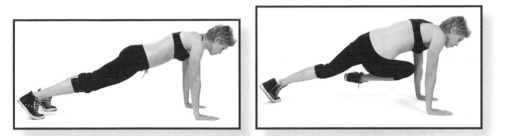

Elbow-to-Knee Touch Plank

- Get in a push-up or plank position on the floor.
- Bring in one knee to touch the opposite elbow.
- Go back to the starting position.
- Alternate to the other side.

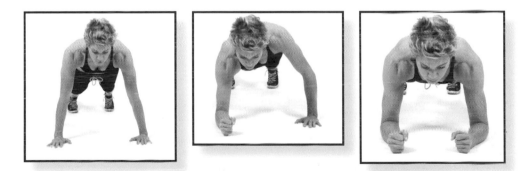

Up-Down Plank

- Get into a push-up position with your hands on the floor a little wider than shoulder-width apart.
- From that position, drop to one elbow, then the other.
- Come back up into the push-up position.

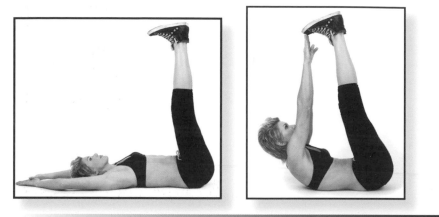

Straight-Leg Toe Touch

- Lie on your back with legs lifted so that they are perpendicular to the floor.
- Crunch upward at your abs and attempt to touch your toes.
- Repeat the exercise for the required number of reps.

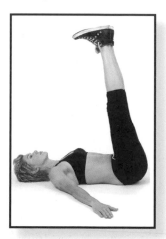

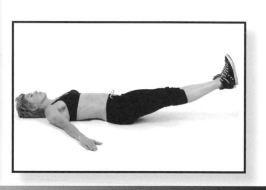

Straight-Leg Drop

- Lie on your back with your legs lifted so that they are perpendicular to the floor and your hands palm-down gripping the floor.
- Slowly lower your legs until they are 2 inches (5cm) from the floor.
- Raise to the starting position.

Cool-Down Stretches

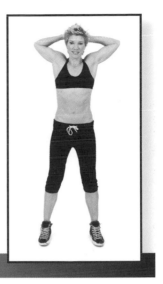

Chest Stretch

- Place your hands behind your head and interlock your fingers.
- Keep your elbows lifted.
- Press your chest forward and your elbows back, getting a good stretch in your chest.

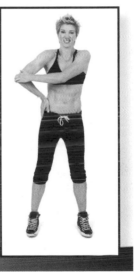

Shoulder Crossover Stretch

- Stand with your feet about shoulder-width apart. Put your right hand on your hip.
- Reach your left arm across your chest. Take your left hand and grab your right elbow. Press your left arm closer to your body and get a good stretch in your left shoulder. Repeat on the other side.

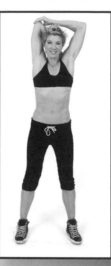

Triceps Stretch

- Stand with your feet about shoulder-width apart.
- Raise your right arm straight overhead. Bend your elbow and place your right palm behind your neck or on the top of your back, wherever you can reach.
- Maintain a straight spine and neck, and do not push your head forward. With your left hand, tug your right elbow slightly to get a good stretch in your triceps muscle.
- Repeat the stretch on the opposite side.

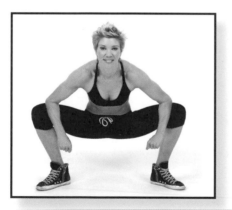

Squat Stretch

- Stand with your legs wider than shoulder-width apart.
- Squat down and hold for a few seconds, getting a good stretch in your inner thighs.

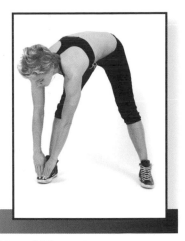

Toe Touch

- Stand with your feet slightly wider than shoulder-width apart.
- Bend at the waist and touch your right toes. Return to start and repeat on the left side. Get a good stretch in your hamstring muscles at the back of your legs.

During each phase of the 10x10 Fitness Program workout, you'll meet weekly training goals and follow an easy plan designed for quick weight loss. Not only will you look better than when you started, but you'll become the confident, high-performing person you were meant to be.

Ideally, you'll want to block out 30 to 45 minutes for your workouts over the next ten days. Bottom line: Get your workout days in no matter when, where, or how.

You can do the 10x10 Program workout at home or at a gym.

Start thinking like an athlete and you will start seeing yourself as attractive, energetic, strong, and in sync with your body. It is the greatest gift you have been given—so start using it!

PART 2

The Program

Now we're at the *fun* part!

The 10x10 Program can change your life. I'm not kidding. It really can.

It's broken down into three phases, each lasting ten days. Each ten-day phase features:

- Superstar Foods
- Grocery lists
- A specific diet for each phase
- A specific workout for each phase

As you progress through each phase, you'll not only experience weight loss, but also:

- Feel better physically, mentally, and emotionally
- Find it easier to eat a healthy, balanced diet
- Exercise more efficiently, with faster results

Your body has been craving these foods for a lifetime. Keep your eye on the prize and focus on having a great attitude of excitement. Start each day with a sense of purpose: to eat healthily and exercise.

I strongly believe that *can't* means "won't." If you won't do it now, when will you? If you won't allow yourself a life of happiness and self-empowerment, who will?

When you commit to the 10x10 Program, each day will get better. It will get easier to eat healthy foods and exercise to your maximum potential. After you complete the first phase of the program, you'll find the second and third phases so much easier, simply because you've committed yourself to a new path.

It's an amazing journey, and I'm so glad you've chosen me to take it with you!

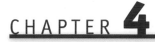

Phase 1: The First 10 Days

The 950-Calorie Diet

OKAY, I KNOW YOU ARE DYING TO GET STARTED.
Now you're going to learn all the secret Superstar Foods that are the very
best for preventing weight gain and encouraging fat loss, increasing
energy, recharging your metabolism, improving serotonin levels in the
brain, and satisfying cravings. They will switch on the genes that tell
your body to burn more fat; eating them can be as effective as taking
a magic pill. You will see a positive effect within 24 hours. That's right,
I am telling you that you can change your body's chemistry that fast!
Given the high level of nutrients in these foods, your body will change
gears and start the process of operating at a higher level.

In my last book, *This Is Why You're Fat*, I gave you recipes that could
all be prepared in under ten minutes. I also provided non-cook options.
Most readers really loved the "non-cook" portion of the diet, for the
same reason I do: I don't have time to cook! I love the idea that if I go to
an organic market, and I keep my calories and sugar down to what I
need per serving, I can just mindlessly toss foods into my cart, and
then—yes, I'm admitting to it—microwave. You may not be as lazy as me

when it comes to cooking, but the point is, you can be—and still lose weight.

Every ten days, I'll give you the 10x10 grocery list and tell you why your Superstar Foods are working instantly for you and exactly what to eat. You'll follow the same type of food plan every single day—no deviation. Just follow the 10x10 Diet and watch the weight drop off. By Day 7, you will start wanting to switch foods—but sit tight, you have only three more days until the next round. It couldn't be easier—just stock up with my grocery list, then follow my eating plan, and watch the weight drop off. The best way to be a confident leader for yourself is to have a clear understanding of what and why you do something. So here are the Superstar Foods you'll be eating over the next ten days, along with some fun facts about them and why they work!

Phase 1: 10 Superstar Foods

Superstar 1. Apples

Serving Size: 1 medium apple

Apple Facts

Calories	95
Total Fat	0g
Total Carbohydrate	25g
Fiber	4.4g
Protein	0.5g

SuperSTAR Ingredient: Pectin

Fat-Burning Power:

Pectin fiber in apples slows digestion and controls appetite. One apple has the same amount of fiber that is contained in a bowl of bran cereal. Also, the pectin contained in apples supplies the body with galacturonic acid, which is a substance that decreases the body's insulin needs. Insulin is a fat-forming hormone, so you want to keep it normalized in your body.

Good Medicine:

- Apples are full of phytochemicals (plant chemicals) to prevent cancer.
- They contain the flavonoid phloridzin and the mineral boron, which help prevent osteoporosis.
- They also contain quercetin, which helps prevents Alzheimer's disease.

Fun History:

Archaeologists have found evidence that humans have been enjoying apples since at least 6500 BC. In 400 BC, the Greek physician Hippocrates was the first to recommend apples to cure ailments.

Superstar **2. Avocados**

Serving Size: ¼ of a whole avocado

Avocado Facts

Calories	80
Total Fat	7.37g
Total Carbohydrate	1.5g
Fiber	1g
Protein	1g

SuperSTAR Ingredient: Monounsaturated Fat

Fat-Burning Power:

Monounsaturated fats like those found in avocados help increase your metabolism, allowing your body to burn fat more quickly. Better yet, eating monos keeps your belly skinny. That's because, when your metabolism increases, fat cells in the abdomen are the quickest to give up their fat. Research has shown that women who switched to a 1,600-calorie, high-monounsaturated-fat diet shed a third of their belly fat in a month. Avocados are a nutrient-rich fruit that I use in place of mayo and cheese to really give foods flavor!

Good Medicine:

- Avocados are packed with nearly 20 vitamins, minerals, and phytonutrients that fight chronic and age-related diseases.

- They're a good source of beta-sitosterol, a phytochemical that helps lower blood cholesterol.
- And they're full of glutathione, the most powerful antioxidant, which protects cell DNA from free radicals. This delays aging as well as helping to prevent cancer.

Fun History:

Avocados were once a luxury food reserved for the tables of royalty.

Superstar **3. Broccoli**

Serving Size: 175g (6oz), cooked or raw

Broccoli Facts

Calories	31
Total Fat	0.4g
Total Carbohydrate	6g
Fiber	2.4g
Protein	2.6g

SuperSTAR Ingredient: **Indoles**

Fat-Burning Power:

Broccoli is rich in indoles, food compounds that help reduce bad estrogen. Most people are estrogen-dominant because they consume a lot of processed foods; this makes it super-hard to lose belly fat. Too much estrogen in your body increases fat storage and can block muscle growth. Broccoli is my secret weapon against cellulite. This amazing cruciferous veggie contains alpha-lipoic acid, which helps prevent the hardening of collagen caused by sugar, and also decreases dimpling.

Good Medicine:

- Broccoli is a fabulous source of bone-building calcium.
- It's high in potassium to prevent hypertension.
- The florets are loaded with beta-carotene, an antioxidant that protects against cancer and heart disease.

Fun History:

Broccoli originated in the eastern Mediterranean and Asia Minor and spread to Italy in the 16th century. Today the average person in the United States eats 4½lb (2kg) of broccoli a year. You're about to blow that number out of the water!

Superstar 4. Chicken Breast

Serving Size: 1/2 breast (about 85g/3oz or what will fit in the palm of your hand)

Chicken Breast Facts

Calories	93
Total Fat	2g
Total Carbohydrate	0g
Fiber	0g
Protein	17g

SuperSTAR Ingredient: Branched-chain amino acids

Fat-Burning Power:

Chicken breasts are high in the three most important branched-chain amino acids (BCAAs): leucine, isoleucine, and valine. BCAAs are absolutely necessary as the building blocks for new muscle growth and repair, but they also provide energy to the muscles. These three amino acids also help your body burn fat, improve your recovery, and reduce your muscle soreness after a workout. They also counteract the effects of the stress hormone cortisol; this in turn decreases your appetite, reduces fat storage, and helps your body use sugar more efficiently.

Good Medicine:

- Chicken breast is a great source of niacin, which helps lower cholesterol.
- It's high in selenium, an antioxidant cancer fighter.
- It can also increase protein synthesis and help prevent protein breakdown.

Fun History:

Heard about the incubators that are used at poultry farms? Well, the prototype appeared about 4,000 years ago, in Egypt, and could hold 10,000 chicks.

Superstar **5. Grapefruit**

Serving Size: ½ medium grapefruit

Grapefruit Facts

Calories	41
Total Fat	0.1g
Total Carbohydrate	10.3g
Fiber	1.4g
Protein	0.8g

SuperSTAR Ingredient: Naringin

Fat-Burning Power:

A 12-week pilot study in the United States, reported in *Chemistry & Industry* magazine, found that eating half a grapefruit three times a day helped 100 obese volunteers lose up to 10 lb (4.5kg) in a few months just by adding it to their existing diet! First, grapefruit lowers levels of insulin, which makes people less hungry and sugar less likely to be metabolized as fat. Second, grapefruit contains naringin, which blocks the uptake of fatty acids into cells to prevent our bodies from effectively using carbohydrates. Grapefruit is nature's extreme fat burner!

Good Medicine:

- Grapefruit is loaded with vitamin C, which helps neutralize the free radicals that can damage cells and cause aging and disease.
- It contains more than 60 phytonutrients, a class of natural antioxidants that help the body in its battle against aging, allergies, infection, cancer, and heart disease.
- It's high in pectin, a fiber that helps the body to maintain healthy cholesterol.

Fun History:

The variety of grapefruit popular in the United States was discovered in Barbados. It was brought to Florida in the 1800s. The grapefruit is believed to be a mutation of the pomelo and orange and was referred to as "the forbidden fruit" of Barbados in 1750. It is thought that it got the name *grapefruit* because of the way it grows, hanging in clusters like grapes from the tree.

Superstar **6. New Potatoes**

Serving Size: 3 small potatoes

New Potato Facts

Calories	93
Total Fat	0g
Total Carbohydrate	20.2g
Fiber	3.1g
Protein	1.6g

SuperSTAR Ingredient: **Resistant Starch**

Fat-Burning Power:

Resistant starch is a type of carb that is not digested by the body, and thereby delivers some of the same appetite-suppressing benefits as fiber. The magic of resistant starch goes beyond filling you up. It helps the body burn calories from the fat you eat and the fat you store. Yes, I am saying potatoes are good for you. It's time to welcome them back to your diet—just keep them unloaded!

Good Medicine:

- The resistant starch in potatoes may reduce cancer risks and help control blood sugar levels, thereby reducing the risk of diabetes.
- They're high in potassium to help lower blood pressure.
- And they're rich in vitamin C, an antioxidant that defends the body against heart disease, cancer, and other chronic disease.

Fun History:

Although you probably won't find them on the menu at your favorite Chinese restaurant, the country that actually grows more potatoes than any other is . . . China!

Superstar 7. Porridge

Serving Size: 125g (4½oz) cooked

Porridge Facts

Calories	74
Total Fat	1.2g
Total Carbohydrate	12.7g
Fiber	2g
Protein	3.1g

⭐ *SuperSTAR Ingredient:* **Beta-glucan**

Fat-Burning Power:

The soluble fiber in porridge is called beta-glucan. It acts like a sponge in the stomach, absorbing fat and cholesterol and flushing them out of the system. Porridge is perfect for breakfast because it is a slow-burning carb that lowers insulin levels and increases fat burning during the day. Eating slow-digesting carbs in the morning burns more fat during exercise. The insoluble fiber in oats aids digestion and promotes regularity.

Good Medicine:

- The insoluble fiber in porridge is an anti-cancer agent. Cancer-fighting properties are due its ability to reduce toxicity by attacking bile acids in the body.
- Oats contain iron, vitamins B and E, selenium, and zinc to increase memory.
- Phytochemicals in oats help fight hormonal diseases like breast, prostate, and ovarian cancer.

Fun History:

Ancient Greeks and Romans considered oats to be "barbarian" food and fed them only to animals. It was oat-eating Germanic tribes who later defeated the Romans, resulting in the fall of the Western Roman Empire. Today Americans buy enough porridge to fill 346 million bowls each year.

Superstar **8. Spinach**

Serving Size: 100g (3½oz) cooked

Spinach Facts

Calories	20
Total Fat	0g
Total Carbohydrate	3.4g
Fiber	2g
Protein	2.5g

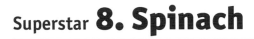 **SuperSTAR Ingredient: Beta-ecdysterone**

Fat-Burning Power:

Popeye was on to something. This power green is one of the richest sources of beta-ecdysterone, a phytochemical that protects plants from insects but has powerful anabolic properties in humans. It boosts protein synthesis, the process that makes muscle grow.

Spinach is also a super source of many other nutrients that are important for muscle building and strength. It's rich in glutamine, the amino acid that is highly important for muscle growth, immune function, and gastrointestinal health. Spinach also contains octacosanol, a compound that has the ability to increase muscle strength.

Good Medicine:

- Spinach is rich in eye-protective lutein, which is the antioxidant found in the highest concentration in the eyes.
- It's also rich in glutathione, which has a detoxifying effect on the liver.
- Spinach is useful in the fight against cancer thanks to all the antioxidants and phytochemicals it contains.

Fun History:

After the introduction of Popeye the Sailor in the comics in 1929, spinach sales rose by about a third. Kids later rated it as their third favorite food, behind turkey and ice cream. (Kids must have been a little healthier back then!)

Superstar 9. Sprouts, Alfalfa

Serving Size: 100g (3½oz)

Sprout Facts

Calories	10
Total Fat	0.2g
Total Carbohydrate	1.3g
Fiber	0.8g
Protein	1.3g

SuperSTAR Ingredient: **Vitamin C**

Fat-Burning Power:

Alfalfa sprouts provide the antioxidant vitamin C, which is known for speeding up the metabolism and burning fat. Sprouts are also low in fat, low in calories, and cholesterol-free. They are full of enzymes that speed up digestion, including proteolytic and amylolytic enzymes. These enzymes digest proteins and carbohydrates. When food is properly digested, it goes directly to your cells to be burned as fuel and is less likely to be packed away as fat.

Good Medicine:

- Sprouts contain canavanine, a protein compound that fights against pancreatic and colon cancers, as well as leukemia.
- They're a superb source of saponins. Saponins help lower fat and reduce bad cholesterol (LDLs, or low-density lipoproteins).
- They keep enzyme activity in the body at a maximum—so that we can stay biologically young and healthy. That is why sprouts can be called "the fountain of youth."

Fun History:

Alfalfa sprouts date back to the 1700s. Sailors on voyages used to consume lots of vitamin-C-rich sprouts to prevent attacks of scurvy.

Superstar **10. Celery**

Serving Size: 3 sticks

Celery Facts

Calories	18
Total Fat	0.2g
Total Carbohydrate	4.1g
Fiber	1.9g
Protein	0.8g

SuperSTAR Ingredient: **Calcium**

Fat-Burning Power:

Raw celery has a high concentration of calcium in a ready-to-use form. So when you eat it, the calcium is sent directly to work. This pure form of calcium ignites your endocrine system, which triggers hormones in your body to begin breaking up accumulated fat buildup.

Good Medicine:

- Celery is high in B vitamins and magnesium, which have a calming effect on the nervous system and encourage weight loss by reducing cravings for sweets.
- It lowers blood pressure due to compounds known as phthalides.
- It's rich in heart-healthy vitamin C and folate for beautiful skin.

Fun History:

While it's not known who first cultivated celery, it has been around for almost 3,000 years. The ancient Greeks and Romans used celery as a medicine and not as a food. Celery was also used by the ancient Greeks as an award in sports contests.

Two Superstar Beverages

Green Tea

The 10x10 Diet suggests that you mix one bag of decaf green tea with your favorite herbal fruit tea bag at night. Most people have something called oral fixations, which compel you to snack when you are bored, mainly at night. If you drink tea—decaf or regular—you curb that compulsion and get the benefit of catechins—natural compounds that speed up metabolism and trigger the release of fat. Also, catechins are high in polyphenols, which have potent antioxidant and anti-tumor properties. They appear to protect against Alzheimer's disease and other forms of dementia. And green tea contains an amino acid called thiamine that can be quite calming to the brain. I have my tea every night—it helps me relax and celebrate a job well done!

Water Power!

I have given thousands of tips in my career, but the easiest and most effective tip relates to water consumption and metabolism.

Water helps cleanse your liver and kidneys, allowing your body to excrete hormones efficiently. It also tames cravings. A craving is often a sign of plain dehydration, not a cry for food. Drinking 2–3 liters (3½–5 pints) of water a day burns 50 to 75 additional calories and speeds up your metabolism.

When water isn't a regular part of your diet, it can be hard to suddenly make it the centerpiece of your liquid intake. Maybe you get bored drinking water at every meal, or maybe your body is craving the chemicals in the fizzy drinks you used to have.

There are ways to make water taste better, and when it tastes better you're more likely to want to drink more of it. Weight-loss drink mixes are popular and many feature vitamins, minerals, and electrolytes—but what else?

Most contain ingredients such as artificial fillers and processed or artificial sugars, which rob the body of its ability to operate at maximum efficiency for weight loss and general health. I'm not saying that all drink mixes are bad for you. I'm saying that you have to be smart about your choices.

The best plan is to drink water cold for an extra energy boost. Ice-cold water will wake you up in the afternoon just like coffee, because cold water is a metabolic booster. The reason? It may take extra energy for your body to heat it prior to digestion. Sip water throughout your workouts, too. I advise my clients to get a one-liter refillable bottle that's not plastic. It helps you gauge how much you need to drink, plus lets you avoid the bad toxins that are leached from plastic. You can buy these bottles at most grocery stores.

Phase 1: Grocery List

Produce

3 large bags of fresh spinach

3 beefsteak tomatoes

3 avocados

10 small apples

5 grapefruits

2 bags of frozen broccoli

30 new potatoes

40 whole sticks of celery

5 packets of alfalfa sprouts

Dairy Case

2 x 450g (16oz) tubs of low-fat cottage cheese

Whole Grains and Cereal

1 large packet of plain porridge

2 loaves of wholegrain, seeded bread

Poultry

5 skinless, boneless chicken breasts

Other

1-liter water bottles or reusable 1-liter bottle

2 packets of raw or unsalted almonds

2 packets of raw or unsalted walnuts

2 packets of green tea

2 packets of herbal fruit tea

Coffee

Almond milk

Almond butter

1 jar of minced garlic

1 packet of natural stevia leaf sweetner, such as Truvia or
Canderel Green Stevia

1 jar of mustard

1 bottle of extra-virgin olive oil

Suggested Weight-Loss Support

Whey isolate protein powder

A complete multivitamin for complete nutritional support

An omega 3–6–9 supplement for metabolic balance and beauty

Phase 1: The Diet

Breakfast

142 calories

1 cup coffee with 1 Truvia or stevia sweetner and a dash of almond milk

or

1 cup green tea

½ medium grapefruit

60g (2oz) plain porridge with 1 plain walnut

500ml (18fl oz) cold water

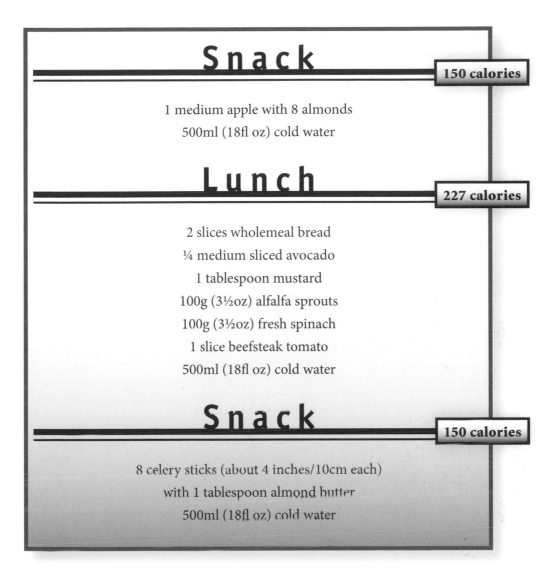

Snack

150 calories

1 medium apple with 8 almonds

500ml (18fl oz) cold water

Lunch

227 calories

2 slices wholemeal bread

¼ medium sliced avocado

1 tablespoon mustard

100g (3½oz) alfalfa sprouts

100g (3½oz) fresh spinach

1 slice beefsteak tomato

500ml (18fl oz) cold water

Snack

150 calories

8 celery sticks (about 4 inches/10cm each)

with 1 tablespoon almond butter

500ml (18fl oz) cold water

Dinner

279 calories

1 precooked chicken breast (175g/6oz) or pan-grilled chicken breast
prepared with ½ teaspoon fresh minced garlic and a
dash of salt and pepper in 1½ teaspoons olive oil
175g (6oz) broccoli (microwaved or steamed)
3 small new potatoes
500ml (18fl oz) cold water

DINNER TIP

*Place all items in a large pan and sauté them together for a major
time-saver. Alternatively, you may grill the chicken and microwave
the broccoli and potatoes. Or buy already-prepared chicken from
the grocery store.*

Post-Dinner

0 calories

1 cup decaf green tea with 1 additional bag herbal fruit tea

Daily Total: 948 calories

As you follow the above plan, make sure you do my 10x10 Fitness
Program along with it to ensure results. It follows in the next chapter.

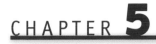

Phase 1: The 10x10 Fitness Program

THE 10X10 FITNESS PROGRAM FEATURES daily workouts that are incredible fat-burning and muscle-toning routines you can do right in your own living room. All you need are three pieces of equipment:

- **A skipping rope.** Any skipping rope will work for the 10x10 daily workouts.
- **A set of light dumbbells** (a pair of 6lb (2.7kg) or 8lb (3.6kg) weights if you're a woman; a pair of 15lb (6.7kg) or 20lb (9kg) weights if you're a man).
- **A set of heavy dumbbells** (a pair of 12lb (5.4kg) or 15lb (6.7kg) weights if you're a woman; a pair of 25lb (11.2kg) or 35lb (15.8kg) weights if you're a man).

Because you're eating roughly 950 calories per day, you don't want to burn more than 200 calories during the Phase 1 10x10 daily workout. So, I have limited your skipping rope rotations. You will be lifting for two sets but only ten reps per exercise. There are a total of 30 exercises you will need to learn throughout the course of the month. Your workouts adjust as your body adjusts. Practice perfecting your form on movements. As you do each move, slow it down to two counts on the way up (the contraction) and two counts on the way down (the lowering portion of the exercise).

I have created a specially designed training sequence based on these key components: weight training to increase muscle tone and resting metabolism, interval cardio to burn fat, and a full-body circuit to help you build lean muscle while destroying body fat. Each component puts into play the intensity principles discussed in chapter 3. Here is an overview.

Days 1, 2, and 3: You will perform ten different exercises broken into two supersets each day. A superset is a combination of different exercises performed back-to-back without a rest period. The workouts will use the following combinations:

- chest, biceps, abs
- shoulders, legs, abs
- back, triceps, abs
- cardio-acceleration

Simply follow each exercise down the list for one long superset, then repeat.

When you lift weights, you build muscle, which is metabolically active tissue. The higher your metabolism, the more fat you will burn. You will be supersetting most exercises. I have incorporated the proven intensity principle of cardio-acceleration in these workout days for a greater fat burn.

Day 4: Interval cardio training—a fat-burning routine to help you achieve better results in less time. This is the most effective and time-efficient way to perform cardio. Basically, it alternates bouts of high-intensity and lower-intensity activity. While the intense bursts burn lots of calories, the recovery periods inbetween draw energy straight from your fat stores, providing a two-pronged fat-burning effect.

Day 5: A full-body circuit routine. When you perform full-body workouts, you increase your fat-burning potential even more in most of your body's muscles, drawing fat into those muscles for use as energy.

Days 6, 7, and 8: You'll repeat the workout from Days 1 through 3:

- chest, biceps, abs
- shoulders, legs, abs
- back, triceps, abs
- cardio-acceleration

Day 9: Interval cardio training again, just like on Day 4.

Day 10: Full-body circuit routine, just like on Day 5.

The 10x10 Daily Workout

Complete one large set by doing this: Perform 2 exercises for chest/2 exercises for biceps/1 cardio-acceleration/2 exercises for chest/2 exercises for biceps/1 cardio-acceleration/2 exercises for abs/1 cardio-acceleration.

Do this straight through for one long superset. **Follow by repeating for a second set**.

For a quick-and-easy reference chart of these exercises, please visit www.jackiewarner.com to download a chart of what you'll need to do for each day of the Phase 1 10x10 workout.

Warm-Up Routine

Prior to every resistance-training workout for the next ten days, perform the following warm-up routine for ten reps each. You can find detailed exercise instructions in chapter 3.

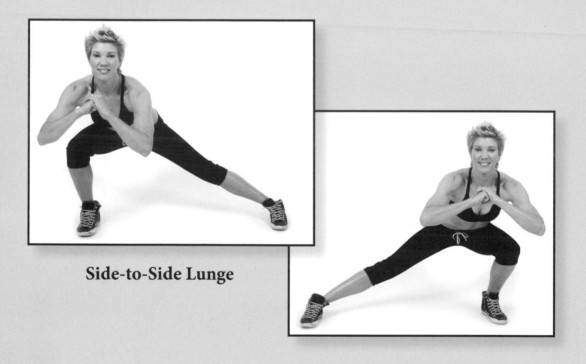

Side-to-Side Lunge

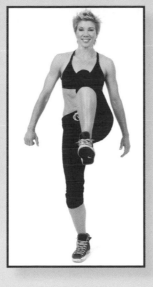

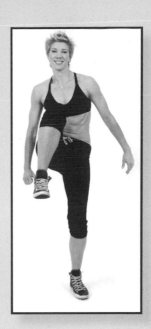

Knee-Up

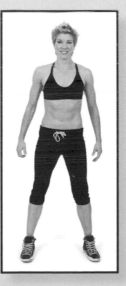

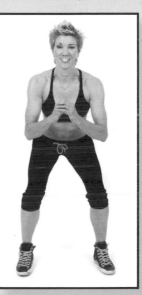

Leg Warm-Up

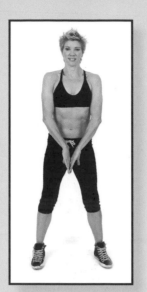 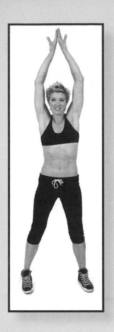

Shoulder Warm-Up

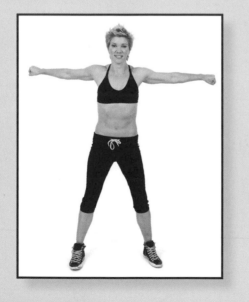

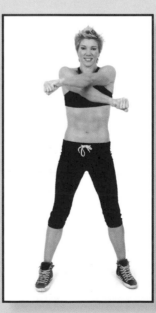

Chest Opener

Cool-Down Stretches

After every resistance-training routine for the next ten days, perform my cool-down stretches. You can find detailed exercise instructions in chapter 3.

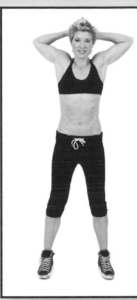

Chest Stretch

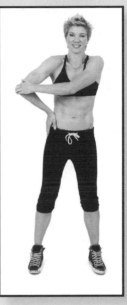

Shoulder Crossover Stretch

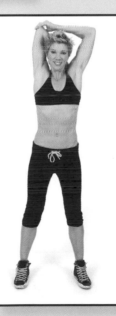

Triceps Stretch

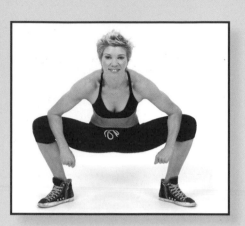

Squat Stretch

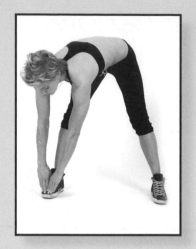

Toe Touch

DAY 1: Chest, Biceps, Abs & Cardio-Acceleration

Exercise	Sets	Reps
Chest		
Flat Press	2	10

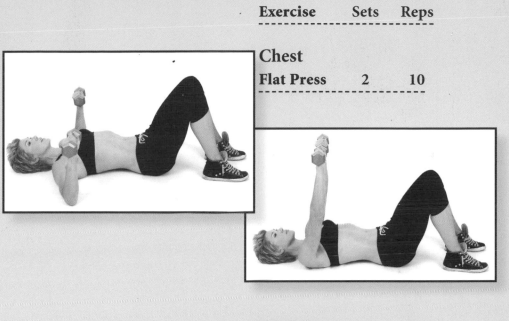

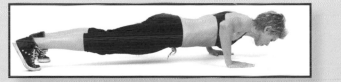

Exercise	Sets	Reps
Push-Up	2	10

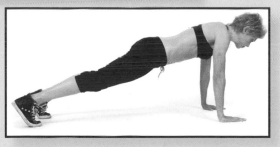

Biceps

Biceps Curl   2   10

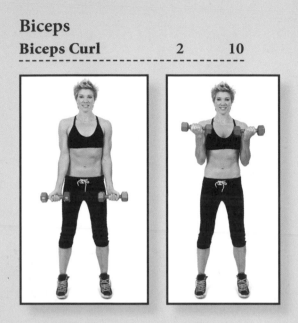

Close Hammer
Curl (squat)   2   10

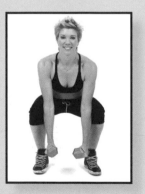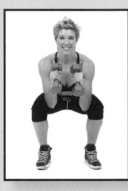

Cardio-Acceleration
100 rotations of skipping rope
1 minute rest

Chest
Incline Press   2   10

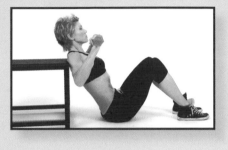 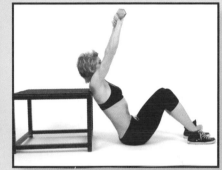

Flat Flye   2   10

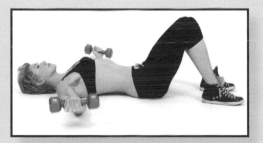 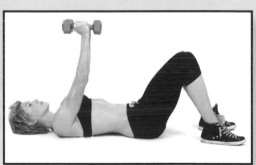

Biceps
Diagonal Curl   2   10

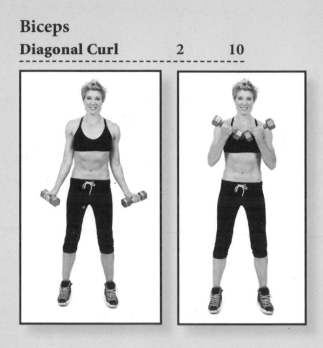

Outer Curl   2   10

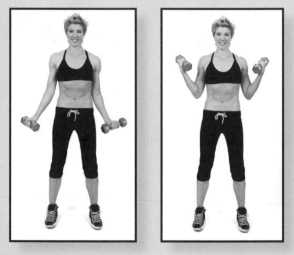

Cardio-Acceleration
100 rotations of skipping rope
1 minute rest

Abs

Bicycle 2 20

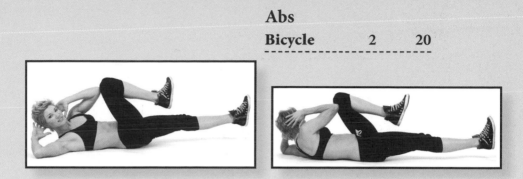

Elbow-to-Knee

Touch Plank 2 20

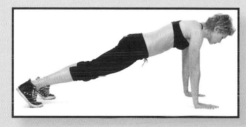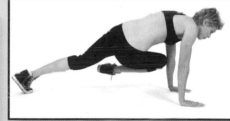

Cardio-Acceleration

100 rotations of skipping rope

1 minute rest

DAY 2: Shoulders, Legs, Abs & Cardio-Acceleration

Shoulders

Exercise	Sets	Reps
Military Press	2	10

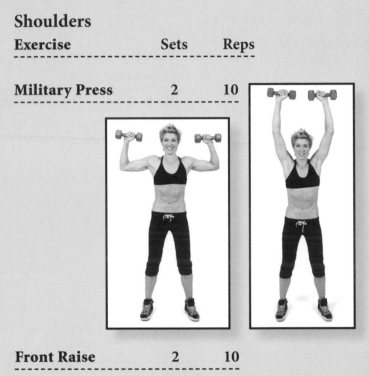

Exercise	Sets	Reps
Front Raise	2	10

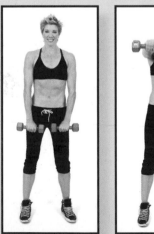

Legs

Deep Squat   2   10

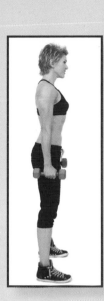

Deadlift   2   10

Cardio-Acceleration
100 rotations of skipping rope
1 minute rest

Shoulders
Hammer Press   2   10

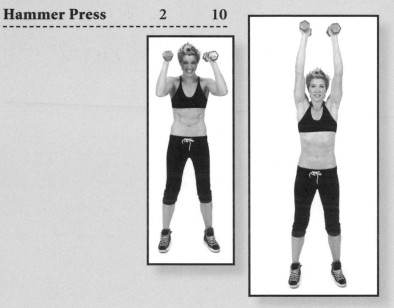

Lateral Raise   2   10

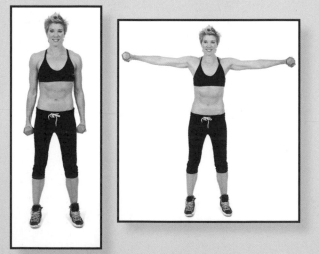

Legs
Sumo Squat   2   10

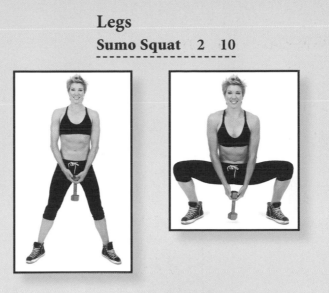

Front Alternating
Lunge   2   20 total, alternating

Cardio-Acceleration
100 rotations of skipping rope
1 minute rest

Abs

Reverse Crunch 2 20

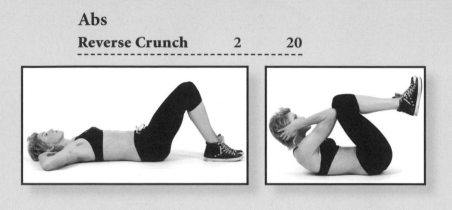

Up-Down Plank 2 20

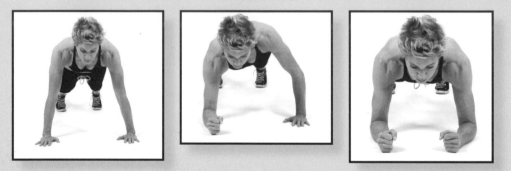

Cardio-Acceleration
100 rotations of skipping rope
1 minute rest

DAY 3: Back, Triceps, Abs & Cardio-Acceleration

Exercise	Sets	Reps
Back		
Bent-Over Wide Row	2	10

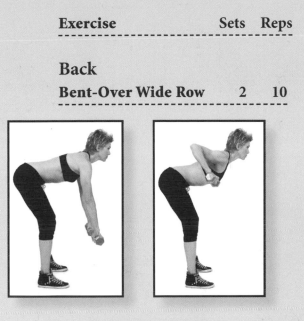

Exercise	Sets	Reps
Reverse-Grip Row	2	10

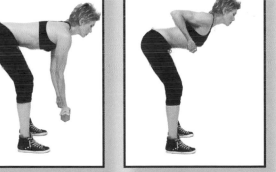

Triceps
Close-Grip Press   2   10

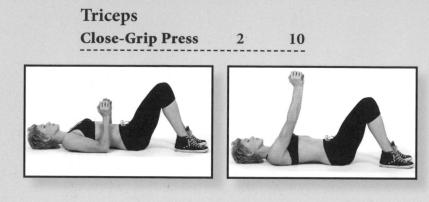

Single Headbanger   2   10

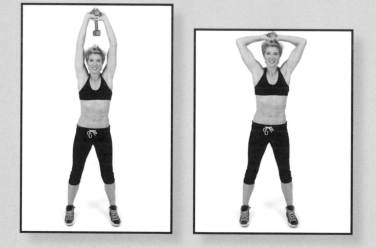

Cardio-Acceleration
100 rotations of skipping rope
1 minute rest

Back

Alternating Row   2   10

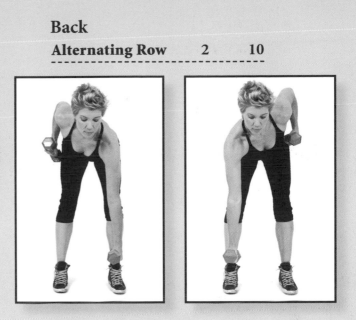

Rear Lateral Raise   2   10

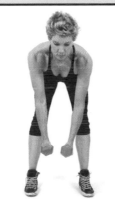
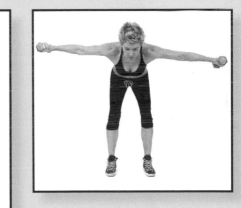

Triceps
Kickback   2   10

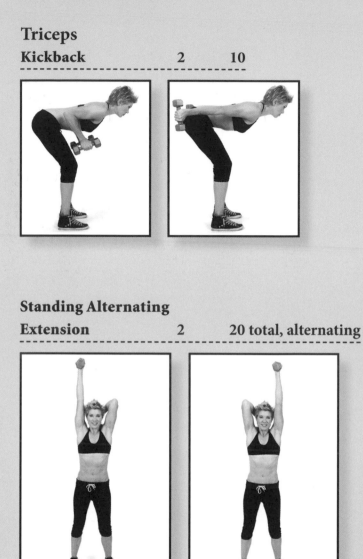

Standing Alternating
Extension   2   20 total, alternating

Cardio-Acceleration
100 rotations of skipping rope
1 minute rest

Abs

Straight-Leg Toe Touch   2   20

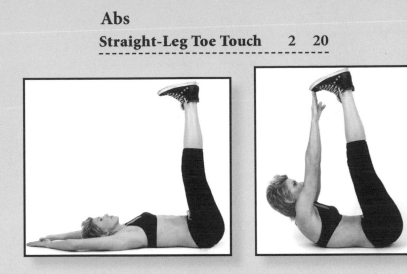

Straight-Leg Drop   2   20

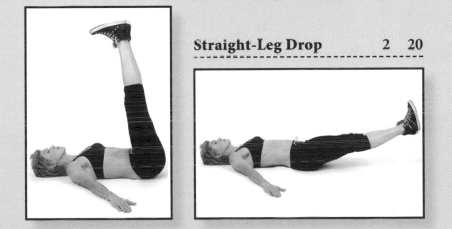

Cardio-Acceleration

100 rotations of skipping rope

1 minute rest

DAY 4: High-Intensity Interval Cardio (HIIT)

Treadmill: 3-minute treadmill jog followed by 1-minute sprint followed by 1-minute cool-down walk equaling 5 minutes. Repeat 5 more times for a total of 30 minutes.

or

Outdoor: 3-minute outdoor jog followed by 1-minute sprint followed by 1-minute cool-down walk equaling 5 minutes. Repeat 5 more times for a total of 30 minutes.

DAY 5: Full-Body Circuit

Rest only as long as it takes to get from one movement to the next.

Exercise	Sets	Reps
Legs		
Deep Squat	2	10

Chest
Flat Press   2   10

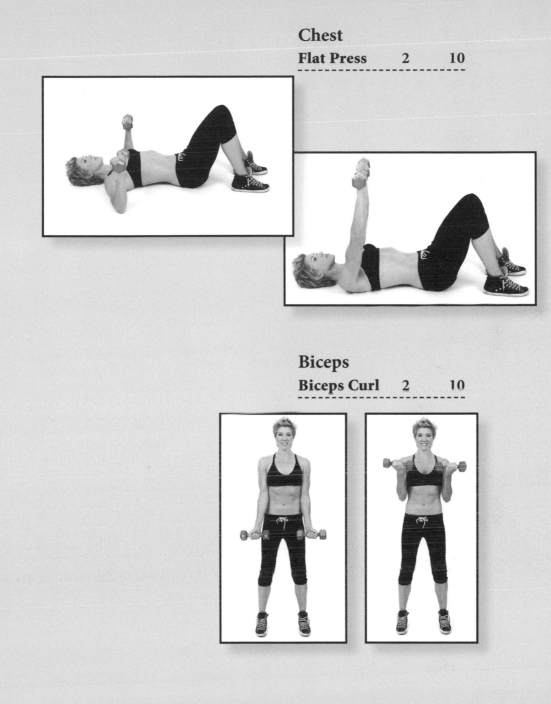

Biceps
Biceps Curl   2   10

Back
Bent-Over Wide Row 2   10

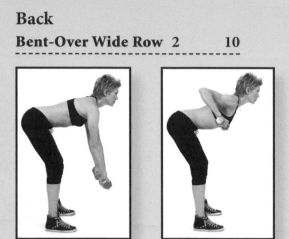

Triceps
Close-Grip Press   2   10

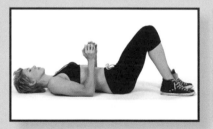 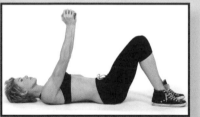

Shoulders

Military Press   2   10

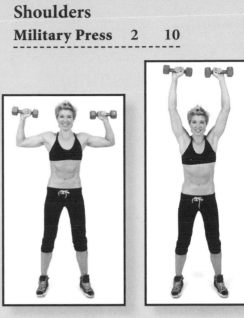

Abs

Bicycle   2   20

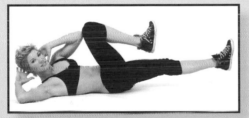
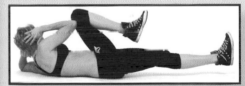

DAY 6: Chest, Biceps, Abs & Cardio-Acceleration

Exercise	Sets	Reps

Chest

Flat Press 2 10

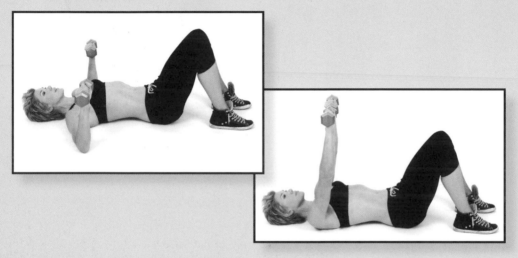

Push-Up 2 10

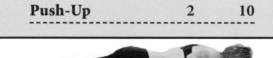

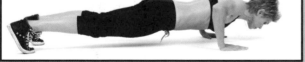

Biceps

Biceps Curl   2   10

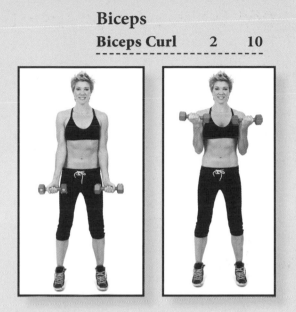

Close Hammer Curl (squat)   2   10

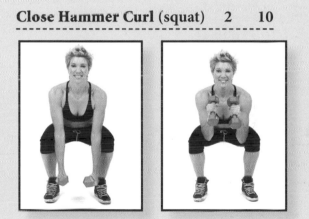

Cardio-Acceleration

100 rotations of skipping rope

1 minute rest

Chest
Incline Press   2   10

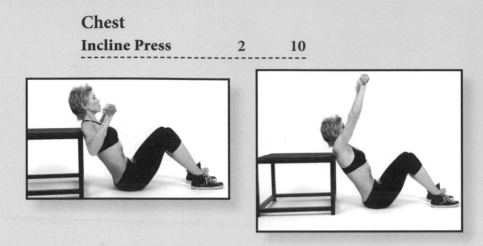

Flat Flye   2   10

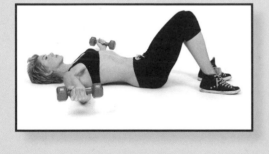

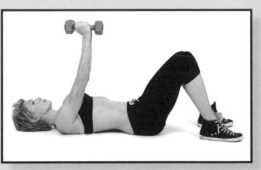

Biceps

Diagonal Curl   2   10

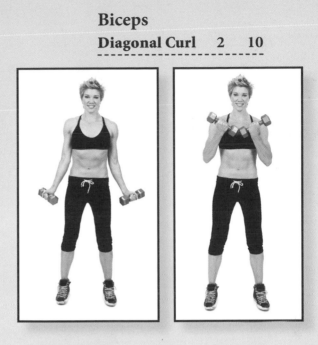

Outer Curl   2   10

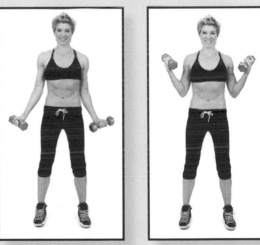

Cardio-Acceleration
100 rotations of skipping rope
1 minute rest

Abs

Bicycle - 2 - - - 20

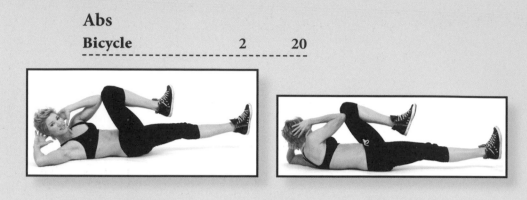

**Elbow-to-Knee
Touch Plank** - - - - - - - - - - - - - - - - - - - 2 - - - 20

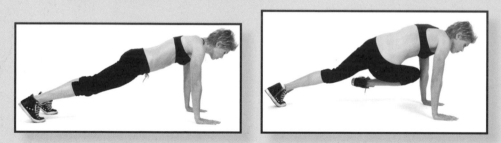

Cardio-Acceleration
**100 rotations of skipping rope
1 minute rest**

DAY 7: Shoulders, Legs, Abs & Cardio-Acceleration

Exercise	Sets	Reps
Shoulders		
Military Press	2	10

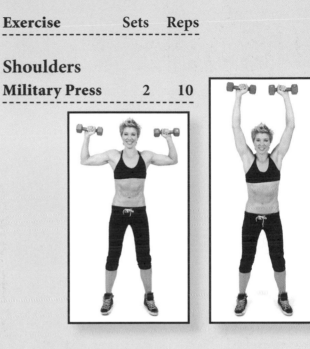

Front Raise	2	10

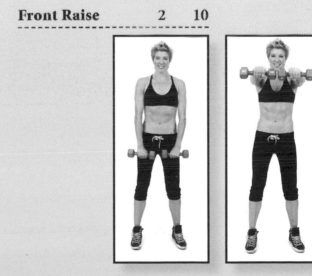

Legs

Deep Squat 2 10

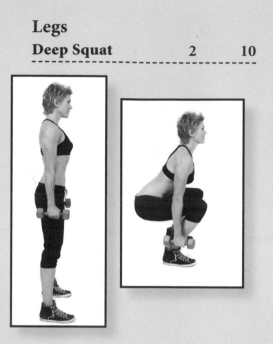

Deadlift 2 10

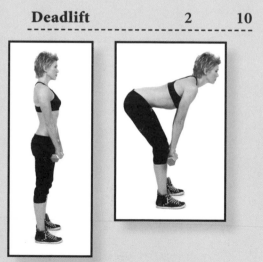

Cardio-Acceleration

100 rotations of skipping rope

1 minute rest

Shoulders
Hammer Press   2   10

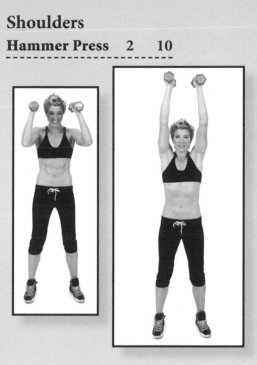

Lateral Raise   2   10

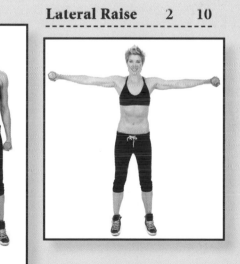

Legs

Sumo Squat 2 10

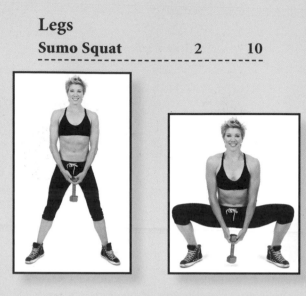

Front Alternating

Lunge 2 20 total, alternating

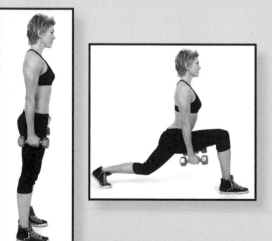

Cardio-Acceleration

100 rotations of skipping rope

1 minute rest

Abs

Reverse Crunch   2   20

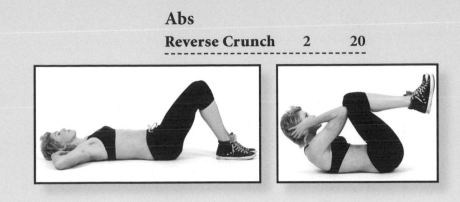

Up-Down Plank   2   20

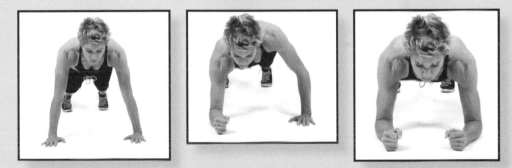

Cardio-Acceleration
100 rotations of skipping rope
1 minute rest

DAY 8: Back, Triceps, Abs & Cardio-Acceleration

Exercise	Sets	Reps

Back
Bent-Over Wide Row 2 10

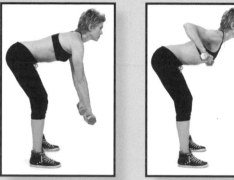

Reverse-Grip Row 2 10

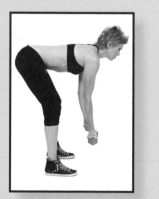 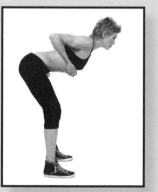

Triceps

Close-Grip Press 2 10

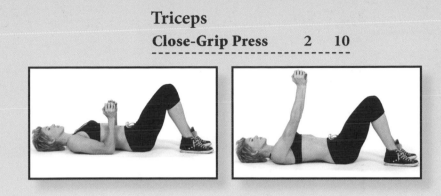

Single Headbanger 2 10

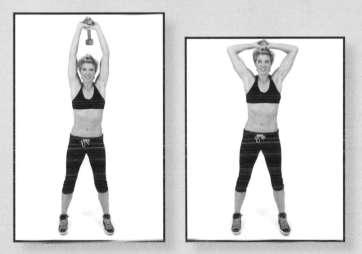

Cardio-Acceleration
100 rotations of skipping rope
1 minute rest

Back

Alternating Row   2   10

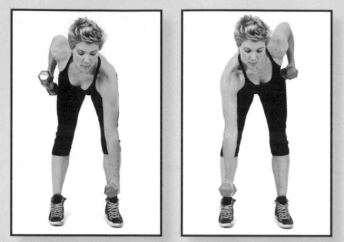

Rear Lateral Raise   2   10

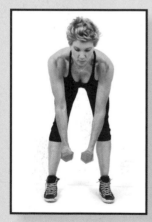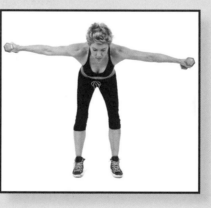

Triceps

Kickback   2   10

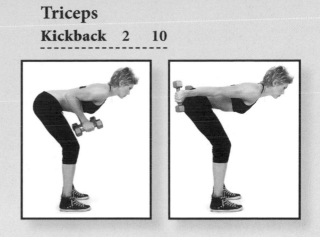

Standing Alternating

Extension   2   20 total, alternating

Cardio-Acceleration

100 rotations of skipping rope

1 minute rest

Abs

Straight-Leg Toe Touch 2 20

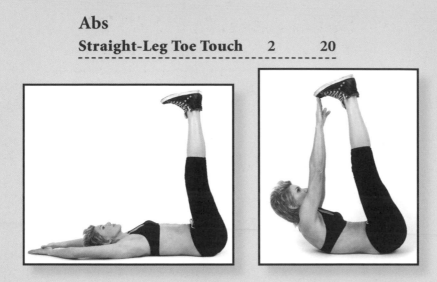

Straight-Leg Drop 2 20

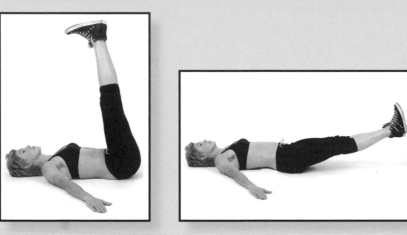

Cardio-Acceleration

100 rotations of skipping rope

1 minute rest

DAY 9: High-Intensity Interval Cardio (HIIT)

Treadmill: 3-minute treadmill jog followed by 1-minute sprint followed by 1-minute cool-down walk equaling 5 minutes. Repeat 5 more times for a total of 30 minutes.

or

Outdoor: 3-minute outdoor jog followed by 1-minute sprint followed by 1-minute cool-down walk equaling 5 minutes. Repeat 5 more times for a total of 30 minutes.

DAY 10: Full-Body Circuit

Rest only as long as it takes to get from one movement to the next.

Exercise	Sets	Reps
Legs		
Deep Squat	2	10

Chest

Flat Press   2   10

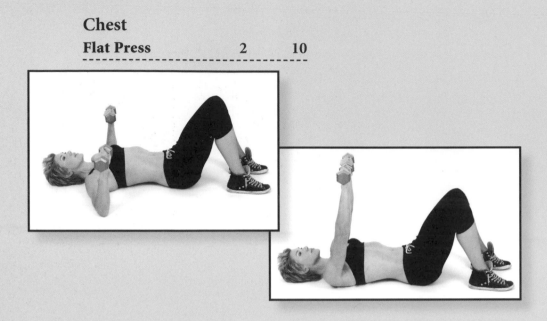

Biceps

Biceps Curl   2   10

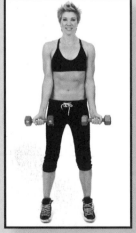 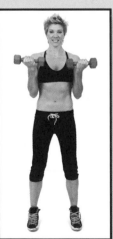

Back
Bent-Over Wide Row   2   10

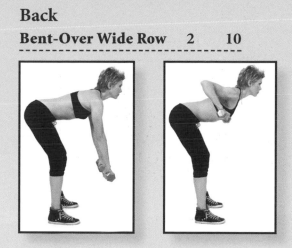

Triceps
Close-Grip Press   2   10

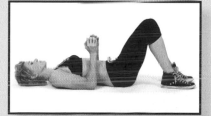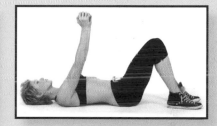

Shoulders

Military Press   2   10

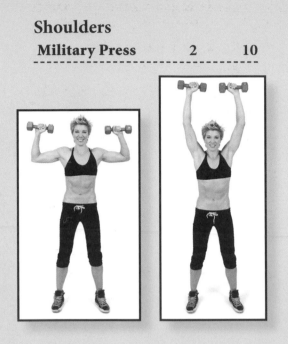

Abs

Bicycle   2   20

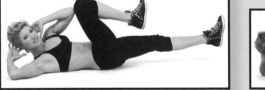 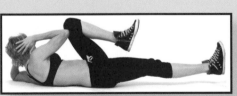

Check your progress on the scales and in the mirror. At this point, you should have met your goal to lose 10lb (4.5kg). If you haven't lost 10lb (4.5kg), don't get discouraged. Become a problem solver. Go back to the weight chart in chapter 2 and ask yourself if you truly had 10lb (4.5kg) to lose—because if you didn't, your body will not want to go under its natural healthy weight. Also, review the 10x10 Diet again and look at portion size. Are you following those portions exactly? If not, then you are consuming more than 950 calories, and weight loss will not be as drastic for you. Continue on to the next ten days and follow the 10x10 Fitness Program fully. You *will* continue to lose weight and get to your goal size, so stay positive and keep going! For those of you who lost 10lb (4.5kg), *congratulations*! You have mastered the 10x10 Program and are ready to move on to maintenance in part 3—or, if you need to lose more, to start Phase 2 of the 10x10 Program.

CHAPTER 6

Phase 2: The Second 10 Days

The 1,200-Calorie Diet

WELCOME TO THE SECOND TEN DAYS. I hope you've weighed yourself already and observed that it is possible to lose up to 10lb (4.5kg) in ten days. Now I know you're fired up to continue.

But before you launch into this part of the diet, I want you to reward yourself—just make sure that reward isn't food or you'll erase all your great work. Think about getting a piece of jewelry, having friends over for a movie or games night, or having a spa day. It is so important to mark positive events in your life. If you don't want to spend money, then soak in a bubble bath, read a great book, listen to music, or take a full afternoon for yourself. In other words, give yourself a break. Celebrate the first 10lb (4.5kg) lost, even if you need to lose more. This will take you to a new level of motivation and self-confidence.

Now here's the 10x10 Diet for the second ten days, along with the ten Superstar Foods I'm emphasizing during this phase. Get familiar with the plan and follow it exactly.

Phase 2: 10 Superstar Foods

Superstar 1. Asparagus

Serving Size: 5 large spears

Asparagus Facts

Calories	40
Total Fat	0.4g
Total Carbohydrate	7.4g
Fiber	3.6g
Protein	4.3g

⭐ SuperSTAR Ingredient: Asparagine

Fat-Burning Power:

Asparagine is an amino acid that helps rid the liver of toxins. The liver is the number one organ responsible for metabolizing fat. Keeping the liver clean will intensify weight-loss results.

Good Medicine:

- Asparagus provides a massive hit of vitamin K, which forms strong bones and keeps the heart healthy.
- It's loaded with folic acid and helps prevent changes to DNA that can cause cancer.
- It contains rutin, a bioflavonoid that has a strong anti-inflammatory effect. Focusing on anti-inflammatory nutrients can help fight aging and age-related diseases like heart disease, cancer, and Alzheimer's. Chronic inflammation can make you look old before your time!

Fun History:

Asparagus has been prized for its medicinal qualities, which were discovered in Greece more than 2,000 years ago. A recipe for preparing asparagus can be found in the oldest surviving cookbook in the world.

Superstar **2. Brown Rice**

Serving Size: 125g (4½oz) cooked

Brown Rice Facts

Calories	108
Total Fat	0.8g
Total Carbohydrate	22.9g
Fiber	1.7g
Protein	2.3g

SuperSTAR Ingredient: **Manganese**

Fat-Burning Power:

Just one cup of brown rice will provide you with 88 percent of your daily manganese. This trace mineral helps produce energy from protein and carbohydrates and is involved in the synthesis of fatty acids, which are important for weight loss, for a healthy nervous system, and in the production of cholesterol, which is used by the body to produce sex hormones. Plus, brown rice keeps nutrients such as fiber and B vitamins intact.

Good Medicine:

- The manganese abundant in brown rice helps your nervous system function and helps the body fight disease-causing free radicals.
- Manganese is needed for collagen formation in skin cells, which is required to keep skin youthful.

- Manganese supports optimal function of the thyroid gland, which helps regulate metabolism.

Fun History:

For the majority of its long history, rice was a staple only in Asia. Not until Arab travelers introduced rice into ancient Greece, and Alexander the Great brought it to India, did rice find its way to other corners of the world.

Superstar **3. Whey Isolate Protein**

Serving Size: 1 scoop

Whey Isolate Protein Facts

Calories	100
Total Fat	2g
Total Carbohydrate	3g
Fiber	0.5g
Protein	18g

SuperSTAR Ingredient: **Leucine**

Fat-Burning Power:

Whey protein, which is derived from dairy products, is a fast-digesting source of amino acids. Whey isolate protein is whey protein that has been microfiltered to create a more pure—and more effective—nutrition source. One amino in particular, leucine, a branched-chain amino acid, helps prevent muscle loss, along with triggering greater loss of belly fat. It works its fat-burning magic by stimulating biochemical processes within muscle cells that result in growth and spike levels of hormones that drive other amino acids into muscle cells. Leucine also takes energy from rich fat cells and gives it to undernourished muscle tissue. Whey protein contains more leucine than milk protein, egg protein, or soy protein.

Good Medicine:

- Whey protein helps deliver more oxygen, nutrients, and muscle-building hormones to your muscles, which provides you with more energy during workouts.
- It enhances the immune system by raising the body's levels of glutathione, a powerful antioxidant produced by the body to protect cells and neutralize toxins.
- It helps prevent age-related bone loss.

Fun History:

In 1749 a patient, who could not be cured by his doctors went to the Swiss mountain village of Gais and was healed by drinking whey on a daily basis. Word spread and people flooded to Gais to benefit from the miraculous properties of whey.

Superstar **4. Carrots**

Serving Size: 10 baby carrots

Carrot Facts

Calories	35
Total Fat	0.1g
Total Carbohydrate	8.2g
Fiber	1.8g
Protein	0.6g

SuperSTAR Ingredient: **Beta-Carotene**

Fat-Burning Power:

Carrots are full of beta-carotene, a form of vitamin A that starts a fat-flushing reaction in your system. This reaction will literally wash out fat and waste quickly.

Carrots have a cleansing effect on the liver. They also stimulate digestion and act as a mild diuretic to fight water weight.

Good Medicine:

- Beta-carotene—a building block of vitamin A—is important for vision and cell structure.
- Carrots are a good source of potassium for cardiovascular health.
- They're also a great source of fiber for digestive health.

Fun History:

The ancient Greeks called the carrot a *philtron*, which translates to "love charm." They believed the carrot made both men and women more amorous. Hippocrates recommended that women eat carrot seeds to prevent pregnancy.

Superstar 5. Cottage Cheese, Low-Fat 1 Percent

Serving Size: 50g (2oz)

Cottage Cheese Facts

Calories	41
Total Fat	0g
Total Carbohydrate	1.5g
Fiber	0g
Protein	7g

SuperSTAR Ingredient: Casein

Fat-Burning Power:

Cottage cheese is packed with casein, a slow-digesting protein that has a high content of calcium for weight loss. It helps boost muscle-building testosterone, which will allow you to tone on a low-calorie diet. Also, a serving of 1 percent cottage cheese has more protein and less fat than a serving of lean beef or chicken.

Good Medicine:

- Cottage cheese is high in calcium to prevent osteoporosis.
- It's a good source of the amino acid tryptophan, a natural relaxant.
- An easily digested protein source, it can keep blood sugar levels even, especially when combined with fruit as a snack.

Fun History:

The term *cottage cheese* is believed to have originated in the 19th century when the cheese was usually made in cottages from any milk left over after churning butter.

Superstar 6. Peanut Butter, Sugar-Free All-Natural

Serving Size: 1 tablespoon

Peanut Butter Facts

Calories	105
Total Fat	8g
Total Carbohydrate	3g
Fiber	1g
Protein	4g

SuperSTAR Ingredient: Omega-6 fatty acids

Fat-Burning Power:

The omega-6s are essential fatty acids, which means they're not manufactured by the body and must be obtained through the diet. They trigger fat burning instead of fat storage by boosting the metabolism through fueling the burning of brown adipose tissue, a type of fat commonly dormant in overweight people. Peanut butter is also fairly high in two other fat burners: protein and monounsaturated fat. Just make sure you eat natural butters in the raw form, which contains no nasty trans fats.

Good Medicine:

- The protein in peanut butter provides a concentrated source of energy.
- The soluble fiber in peanuts works to control blood glucose and prevents saturated fat from entering the bloodstream.
- Peanut butter is loaded with the amino acid arginine, which may relax blood vessels for better blood pressure control.

Fun History:

The peanut originated South America as far back as 950 AB. The Inca were known to have made peanuts into a paste during this time, probably the very first peanut butter.

Superstar **7. Sweet Red Peppers**

Serving Size: 1 medium pepper

Sweet Pepper Facts

Calories	33
Total Fat	0.3g
Total Carbohydrate	7.5g
Fiber	2.8g
Protein	1.4g

SuperSTAR Ingredient: **Lycopene**

Fat-Burning Power:

Lycopene—the cancer-preventing red pigment—is also a fat burner. It stimulates the body to use fatty acids for energy instead of storing them as fat.

Good Medicine:

- Red peppers are packed with bioflavonoids, which help heal blood vessels.
- They're rich in beta-carotene and selenium for a strong immune system.
- Vitamin C in this powerhouse veggie helps build collagen, a protein that helps keep skin from sagging (which causes ugly cellulite).

Fun History:

Christopher Columbus gave this vegetable the misleading name *pepper* (*pimiento* in Spanish) after he brought the plant back to Europe. The misnomer was used because he thought it belonged to the black pepper family.

Superstar **8. Onions**

Serving Size: 1 small onion

Onion Facts

Calories	29
Total Fat	<0.1g
Total Carbohydrate	7.1g
Fiber	1g
Protein	0.6g

SuperSTAR Ingredient: **Chromium**

Fat-Burning Power:

Some of the hottest weight-loss supplements are chromium or contain it in some form. But you don't necessarily have to take chromium supplements. You can get this mineral from onions. Among the benefits of chromium are increased energy, better glucose metabolism (proper burning of sugar in the body), fewer sugar cravings, improved mood and vigor, enhanced lean tissue metabolism, more stamina, and less fatigue.

Good Medicine:

- Sulfur compounds in onions provide anti-cancer capabilities that appear to be potent agents in blocking or suppressing tumor growth.
- Onions contain antioxidant plant pigments that strengthen your mucous membranes and stabilize your immune cells for allergy relief.

- They also contain antibiotics that fight infection, soothe burns, and relieve itchiness.

Fun History:

Onions originated in the area around Iran and were found in the Pyramids in Egypt buried along with the pharaohs. Alexander the Great ordered his troops to eat onions to improve their vitality.

Superstar **9. Blueberries**

Serving Size: 50g (2oz) cup

Blueberry Facts

Calories	42
Total Fat	0g
Total Carbohydrate	11g
Fiber	2g
Protein	0.5g

SuperSTAR Ingredient: **Antioxidants**

Fat-Burning Power:

Antioxidants can increase metabolic function and help you burn fat more efficiently. They also help you manage hunger. Here's how: Environmental toxins damage cell walls. Damaged cell walls prevent nutrients from entering cells. That means cells are malnourished and can't produce energy. To compensate, cell walls send out signals—*Send more food*—and these translate into hunger. We tend to overeat. But antioxidants prevent oxidation and help cell walls repair, so in essence they prevent hunger and keep metabolism as high as possible.

Good Medicine:

- Blueberries are naturally high in ellagic acid, which has been shown to kill certain cancer cells.
- They may help prevent spider veins thanks to their phytochemicals, which strengthen the walls of tiny blood vessels.
- The red pigments, or anthocyanins, in blueberries help your brain maintain its ability to produce dopamine, a chemical that is crucial for memory, coordination, and feelings of well-being, but that declines as you age.

Fun History:

For both Native Americans and early settlers to North America, blueberries were a big part of the diet and also served as medicine. Blueberry juice was used early in the history of the United States to treat illness, coughs, and digestive issues, and as a relaxant during childbirth.

Superstar **10. Salmon, Wild**

Serving Size: 125g (4½oz)

Salmon Facts

Calories	233
Total Fat	14g
Total Carbohydrate	0g
Fiber	0g
Protein	25g

SuperSTAR Ingredient: **Omega-3 fatty acids**

Fat-Burning Power:

Unless you've been stranded on a desert island, you know that salmon is loaded with omega-3 fats. These good fats encourage the body to take glucose from carbs and repartition it, sending it down glycogen-storing pathways rather than fat-storing ones. These fats also protect against muscle breakdown, which can have a significant impact on speeding up your metabolism.

Good Medicine:

- Salmon reduces the risk of coronary heart disease and sudden cardiac death by fighting chronic inflammation.
- It contains selenium for beautiful hair and skin.
- The omega-3 fats in salmon, DHH and EPA, improve mental health and protect against depression.

Fun History:

Salmon spawning journeys can be hundreds, even thousands of miles long. The longest known trip was made by a Chinook salmon. It swam 2,400 miles (4,000km) inland just to spawn! Salmon tend to come back to the same stream in which they were born because they know it's a safe place for their young to grown up.

Phase 2: Grocery List

Produce

- 1–2 onions
- 10 bags of green salad
- 1 bunch of romaine lettuce
- 1 packet of baby carrots
- 10 sweet red peppers
- 20 sticks of celery
- 50 fresh or frozen asparagus
- 10 apples
- Several bunches of watercress

Dairy Case

- 2 x 450g (16oz) tubs of low-fat cottage cheese

Frozen Foods

- 2 packets of frozen blueberries
- 3 bags of frozen spinach

Whole Grains and Cereal

- 1 large packet of plain porridge
- 2–3 packets of wild rice or brown rice, cooked

Poultry

30 slices of free-range chicken deli slices

Fish

10 salmon fillets (see your deli section for prepared fish)

Other

1 jar of sugar-free peanut butter

1 large tub of hummus

1 bottle of low-cal (no more than 50 calories per serving) vinaigrette
    dressing

1 packet of pine nuts

2 packets of green tea

2 packets of herbal fruit tea

Almond milk

Coffee

1 packet of natural stevia leaf sweetner, such as Truvia or
    Canderel Green Stevia

5 lemons (or 1 bottle lemon juice)

1 bottle olive oil

Dill

Suggested Weight-Loss Support

Whey isolate protein powder

A complete multivitamin for complete nutritional support

An omega 3–6–9 supplement for metabolic balance and beauty

Phase 2: The Diet

Breakfast

220 calories

1 cup coffee with 1 Truvia or stevia sweetner and a dash of almond milk

or

1 cup green tea

500ml (18fl oz) cold water

Jackie's Breakfast Smoothie

Blend:

1 scoups whey isolate protein powder

1 teaspoon sugar-free peanut butter

25g (1oz) plain instant uncooked porridge

25g (1oz) mixed frozen berries

25g (1oz) frozen spinach

Dash of water

Snack

150 calories

10 baby carrots with 4 tablespoons hummus

500ml (18fl oz) cold water

Lunch

257 calories

500ml (18fl oz) cold water

Salad of:

3 free-range deli chicken slices

2 sticks celery, sliced

1 slice of onion

1 medium sweet red pepper, diced

140g (5oz) mixed green lettuce leaves

1 tablespoon vinaigrette

1 tablespoon pine nuts

Snack

197 calories

1 medium apple with 100g (3½oz) low-fat cottage cheese

500ml (18fl oz) cold water

Dinner

379 calories

1 pan-grilled salmon fillet prepared with 1 tablespoon lemon juice and ½ teaspoon

dill in ½ tablespoon olive oil or pre-prepared fish from deli section of grocery

5 frozen asparagus stalks, steamed or microwaved

100g (3½oz)wild rice (preferably instant) prepared with salt and pepper

500ml (18fl oz) cold water

DINNER TIP

Place the veggies and fish in a large pan and cook for a major time-saver!

Post-Dinner

1 cup decaf green tea with 1 additional bag herbal fruit tea

Daily Total: 1,203 calories

Up next is your 10x10 Workout for the second ten days. Now that you are in touch with your muscles, you will be increasing the intensity, forcing your body to lean out!

CHAPTER 7

Phase 2: The 10x10 Fitness Program

THE GOOD NEWS IS that your exercises will not change throughout the course of the 10x10 Fitness Program. The key is to master them and combine them in different ways. For the next ten days you are going to follow the same fat-burning exercises, but with different combinations and increased cardio-acceleration. Your interval cardio stays the same, but your full-body circuit will change slightly in variation. Just follow the routine as laid out.

Here's an overview.

Days 11, 12, and 13: You will perform ten different exercises broken into two supersets each day. The workouts will use the following combinations:

- chest, biceps, abs
- legs, shoulders, abs
- back, triceps, abs
- cardio-acceleration

Simply follow each exercise down the list for one long superset, then repeat.

When you lift weights, you build muscle, which is highly metabolically active tissue. The higher your metabolism, the more fat you will burn. You will be supersetting most exercises. I have incorporated the proven intensity principle of cardio-acceleration on these workout days for a greater fat burn.

Day 14: Interval cardio training—a fat-burning routine to help you achieve better results in less time. This is the most effective and time-efficient way to perform cardio. Basically, it alternates bouts of high-intensity and lower-intensity activity. While the intense bursts burn lots of calories, the recovery periods in between draw energy straight from your fat stores, providing a two-pronged fat-burning effect.

Day 15: A full-body circuit routine. When you perform full-body workouts, you increase your fat-burning potential even more in most of your body's muscles, drawing fat into those muscles for use as energy.

Days 16, 17, and 18: You'll repeat the workout from Days 11 through 13:

- chest, biceps, abs
- legs, shoulders, abs
- back, triceps, abs
- cardio-acceleration

Day 19: You'll do interval cardio training again, just like on Day 14.
Day 20: Full-body circuit routine, just like on Day 15.

For a quick-and-easy reference chart of these exercises, please visit www.jackiewarner.com to download a chart of what you'll need to do for each day of the Phase 2 10x10 Workout.

Warm-Up Routine

Prior to every resistance-training routine for the next ten days, perform the following warm-up routine for ten reps each. You can find detailed exercise instructions in chapter 3.

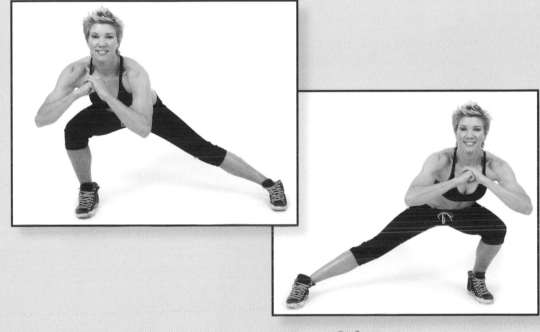

Side-to-Side Lunge

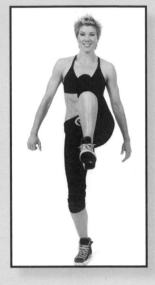
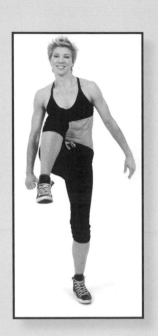

Knee-Up

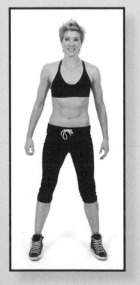
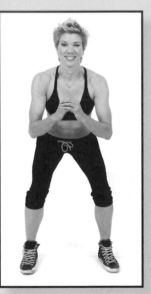

Leg Warm-Up

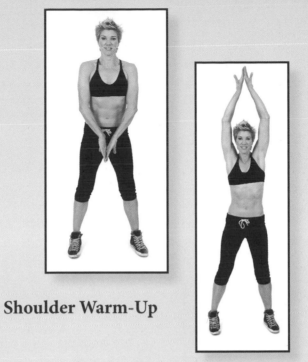

Shoulder Warm-Up

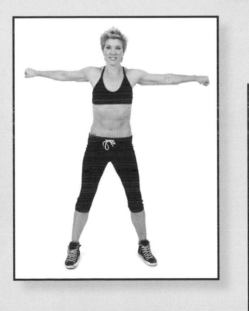

Chest Opener

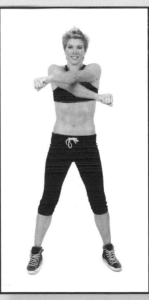

Cool-Down Stretches

After every resistance-training routine for the next ten days, perform my cool-down stretches for 20 seconds each. You can find detailed exercise instructions in chapter 3.

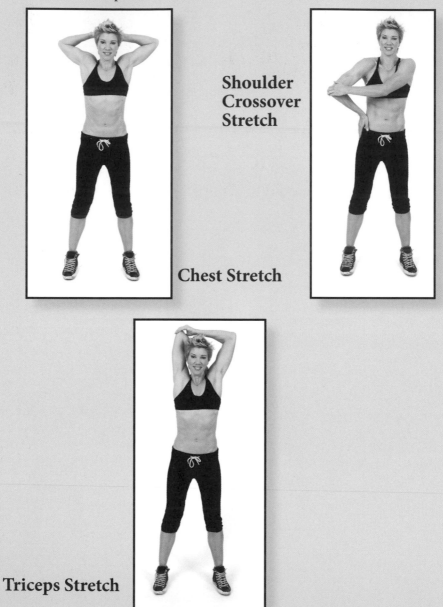

Shoulder Crossover Stretch

Chest Stretch

Triceps Stretch

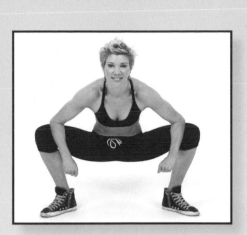

Squat Stretch

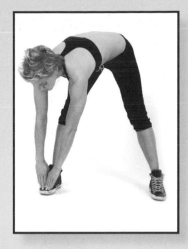

Toe Touch

DAY 11: Chest, Biceps, Abs & Cardio-Acceleration

Exercise	Sets	Reps

Chest

Flat Press	2	10

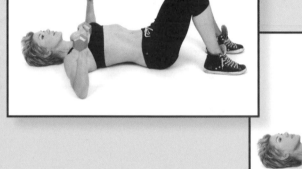

Biceps

Biceps Curl	2	10

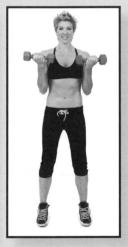

Cardio-Acceleration
200 rotations of skipping rope
1 minute rest

Chest

Incline Press   2   10

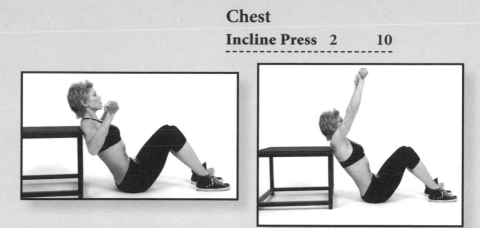

Biceps

Outer Curl   2   10

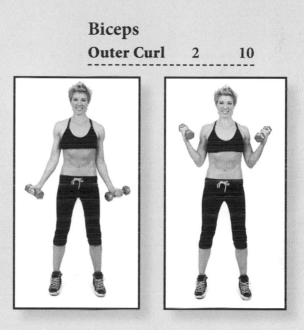

Cardio-Acceleration

200 rotations of skipping rope

1 minute rest

Chest
Flat Flye 2 10

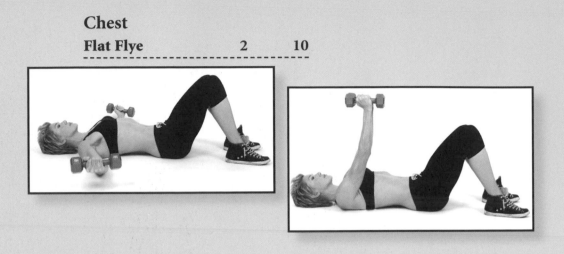

Biceps
Diagonal Curl 2 10

Cardio-Acceleration
200 rotations of skipping rope
1 minute rest

Abs

Straight-Leg Toe Touch 2 20

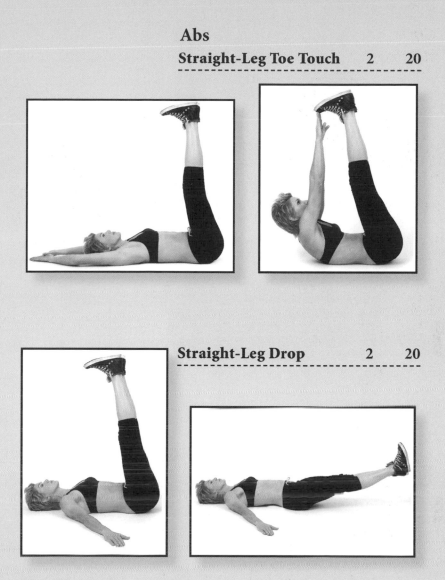

Straight-Leg Drop 2 20

Cardio-Acceleration

200 rotations of skipping rope

1 minute rest

DAY 12: Legs, Shoulders, Abs & Cardio-Acceleration

Exercise	Sets	Reps

Legs
Deep Squat 2 10

Shoulders
Military Press 2 10

Cardio-Acceleration
200 rotations of skipping rope
1 minute rest

Legs
Deadlift 2 10
- -

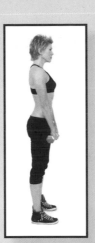
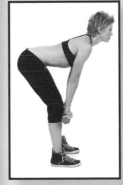

Shoulders
Front Raise 2 10
- -

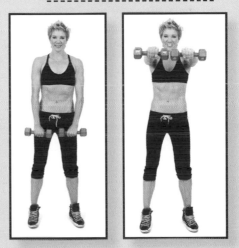

Cardio-Acceleration
200 rotations of skipping rope
1 minute rest

Legs

Sumo Squat   2   10

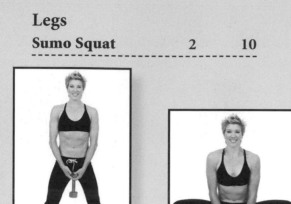

Shoulders

Lateral Raise   2   10

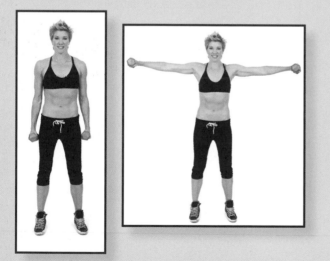

Cardio-Acceleration

200 rotations of skipping rope
1 minute rest

Abs
Up-Down Plank   2   10

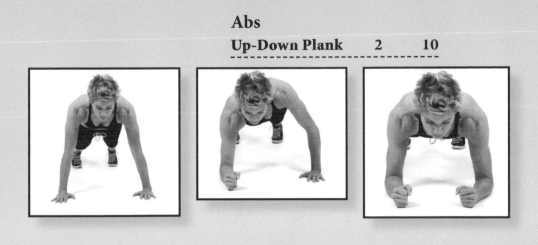

Elbow-to-Knee
Touch Plank   2   10

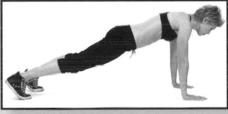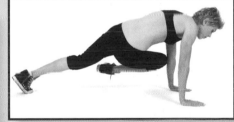

Cardio-Acceleration
200 rotations of skipping rope
1 minute rest

DAY 13: Back, Triceps, Abs & Cardio-Acceleration

Exercise	Sets	Reps

Back
Bent-Over Wide Row 2 10

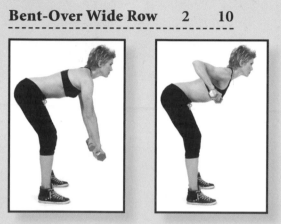

Triceps
Single Headbanger 2 10

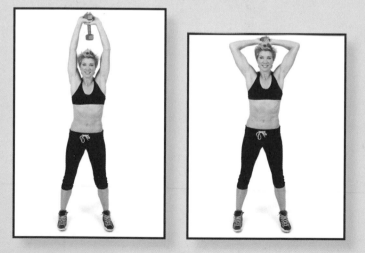

Cardio-Acceleration
200 rotations of skipping rope
1 minute rest

Back
Reverse-Grip Row   2   10

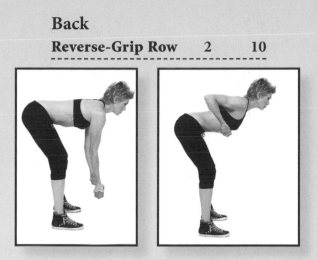

Triceps
Kickback   2   10

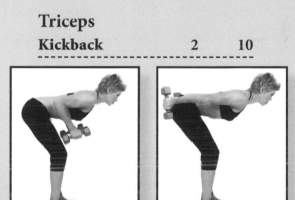

Cardio-Acceleration
200 rotations of skipping rope
1 minute rest

Back
Rear Lateral Raise   2   10

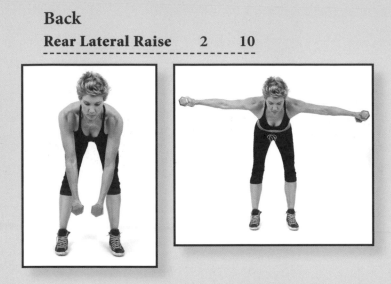

Triceps
Close-Grip Press   2   10

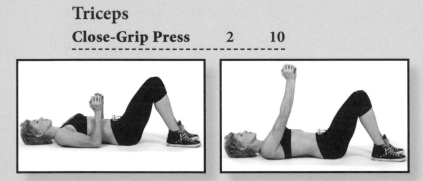

Cardio-Acceleration
200 rotations of skipping rope
1 minute rest

Abs

Bicycle   2   10

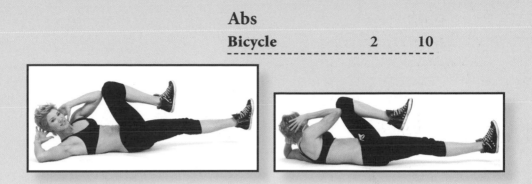

Reverse Crunch   2   10

Cardio-Acceleration
200 rotations of skipping rope
1 minute rest

DAY 14: High-Intensity Interval Cardio (HIIT)

Treadmill: 3-minute treadmill jog followed by 1-minute sprint followed by 1-minute cool-down walk equaling 5 minutes. Repeat 5 more times for a total of 30 minutes.

   or

Outdoor: 3-minute outdoor jog followed by 1-minute sprint followed by 1-minute cool-down walk equaling 5 minutes. Repeat 5 more times for a total of 30 minutes.

DAY 15: Full-Body Circuit

Rest only as long as it takes to get from one station to the next.

Exercise	Sets	Reps
Legs		
Deadlift	2	10

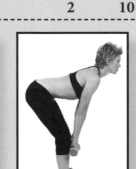

Chest
Incline Press   2   10

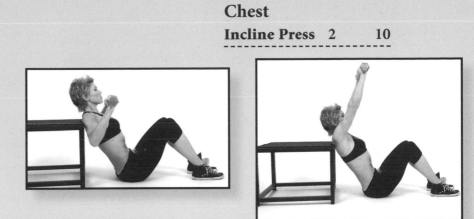

Biceps
Outer Curl   2   10

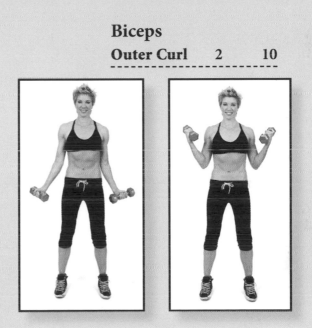

Back

Reverse-Grip Row   2   10

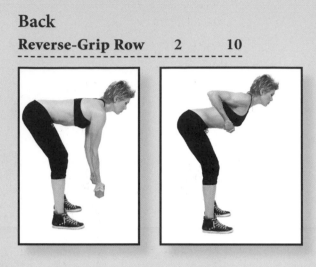

Triceps

Kickback   2   10

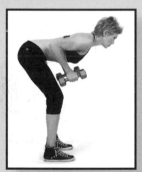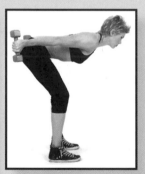

Shoulders

Front Raise   2   10

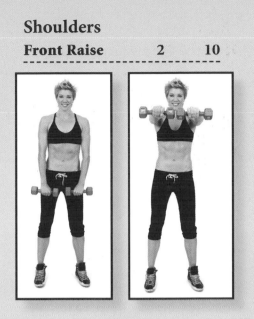

Abs

Reverse Crunch   2   20

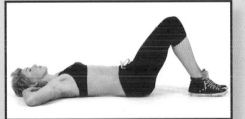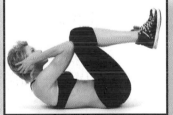

DAY 16: Chest, Biceps, Abs & Cardio-Acceleration

Exercise	Sets	Reps

Chest

Flat Press	2	10

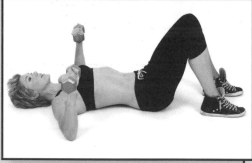

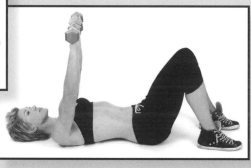

Biceps

Biceps Curl	2	10

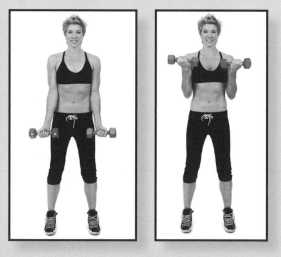

Cardio-Acceleration
200 rotations of skipping rope
1 minute rest

Chest

Incline Press   2   10

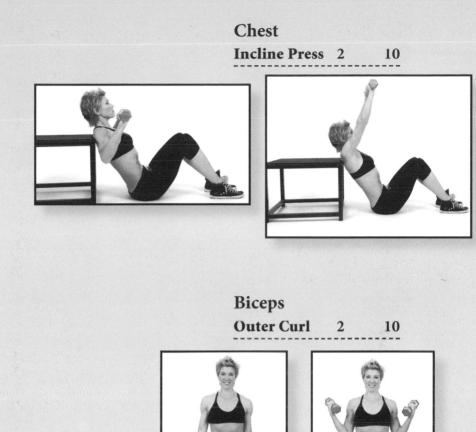

Biceps

Outer Curl   2   10

Cardio-Acceleration

200 rotations of skipping rope

1 minute rest

Chest

Flat Flye   2   10

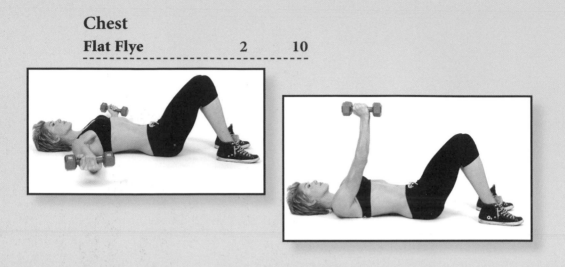

Biceps

Diagonal Curl   2   10

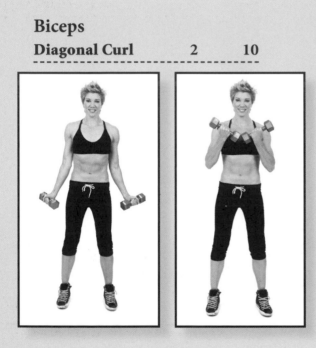

Cardio-Acceleration

200 rotations of skipping rope

1 minute rest

Abs

**Straight-Leg
Toe Touch**   2   10

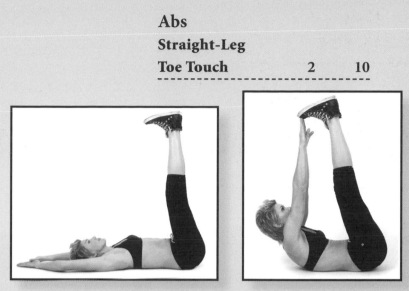

Straight-Leg Drop   2   10

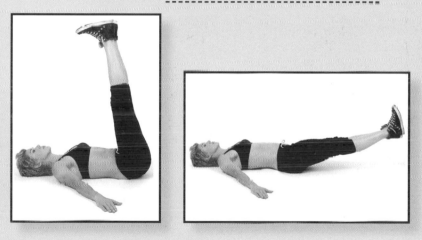

Cardio-Acceleration
**200 rotations of skipping rope
1 minute rest**

DAY 17: Legs, Shoulders, Abs
& Cardio-Acceleration

Legs

Exercise	Sets	Reps
Deep Squat	2	10

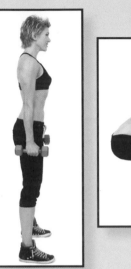
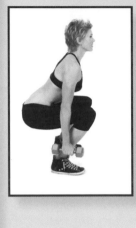

Shoulders

Military Press	2	10

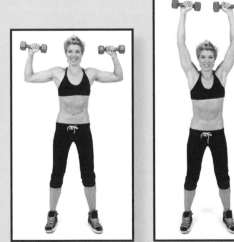

Cardio-Acceleration
200 rotations of skipping rope
1 minute rest

Legs

Deadlift   2   10

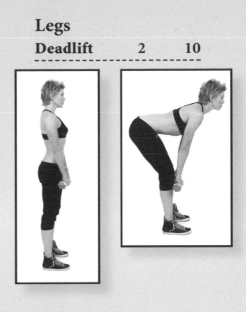

Shoulders

Front Raise   2   10

Cardio-Acceleration

200 rotations of skipping rope
1 minute rest

Legs
Sumo Squat   2   10

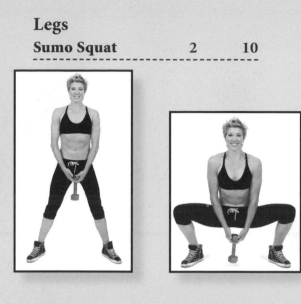

Shoulders
Lateral Raise   2   10

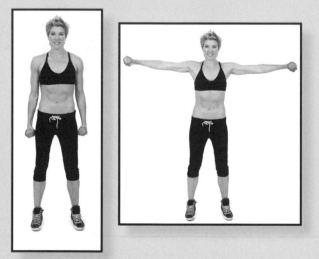

Cardio-Acceleration
200 rotations of skipping rope
1 minute rest

Abs

Up-Down Plank   2   20

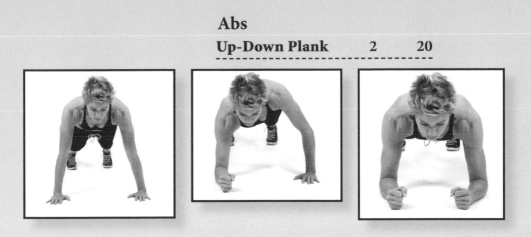

Elbow-to-Knee
Touch Plank   2   20

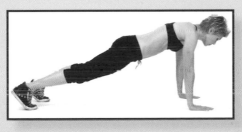
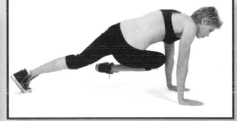

Cardio-Acceleration
200 rotations of skipping rope
1 minute rest

DAY 18: Back, Triceps, Abs & Cardio-Acceleration

Exercise	Sets	Reps

Back
Bent-Over Wide Row 2 10

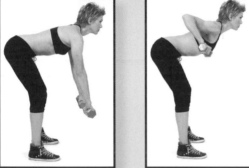

Triceps
Single Headbanger 2 10

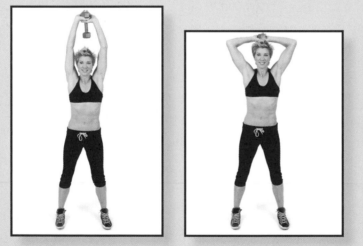

Cardio-Acceleration
200 rotations of skipping rope
1 minute rest

Back
Reverse-Grip Row   2   10

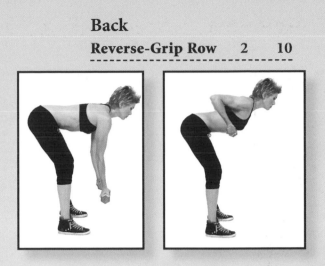

Triceps
Kickback   2   10

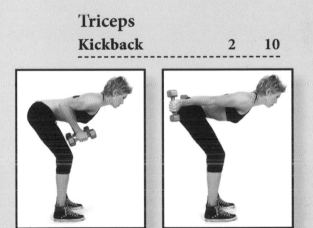

Cardio-Acceleration
200 rotations of skipping rope
1 minute rest

Back
Rear Lateral Raise   2   10

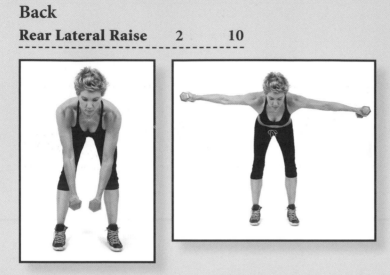

Triceps
Close-Grip Press   2   10

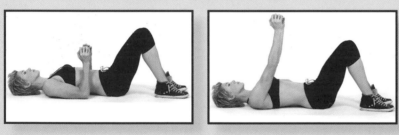

Cardio-Acceleration
200 rotations of skipping rope
1 minute rest

Abs

Bicycle 2 10

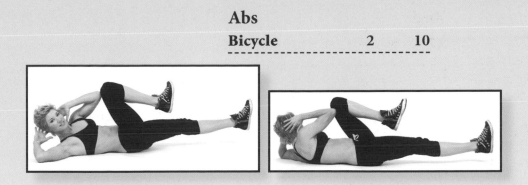

Reverse Crunch 2 10

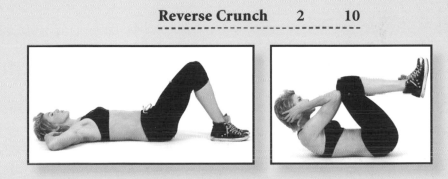

Cardio-Acceleration
200 rotations of skipping rope
1 minute rest

DAY 19: High-Intensity Interval Cardio (HIIT)

Treadmill: 3-minute treadmill jog followed by 1-minute sprint followed by 1-minute cool-down walk equaling 5 minutes. Repeat 5 more times for a total of 30 minutes.

or

Outdoor: 3-minute outdoor jog followed by 1-minute sprint followed by 1-minute cool-down walk equaling 5 minutes. Repeat 5 more times for a total of 30 minutes.

DAY 20: Full-Body Circuit

Rest only as long as it takes to get from one station to the next.

Exercise	Sets	Reps
Legs		
Deadlift	2	10

Chest

Incline Press   2   10

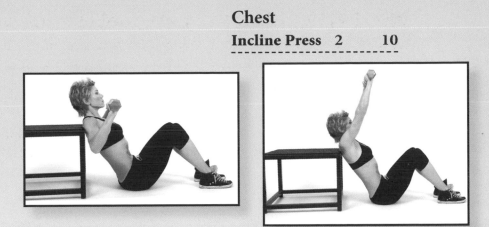

Biceps

Outer Curl   2   10

Back
Reverse-Grip Row   2   10

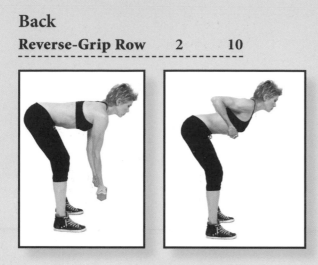

Triceps
Kickback   2   10

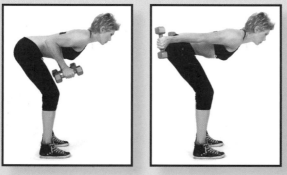

Shoulders

Front Raise   2   10

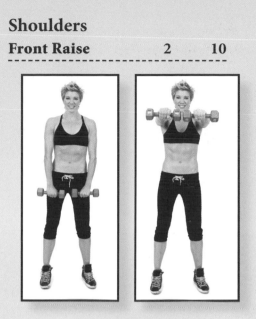

Abs

Reverse Crunch   2   20

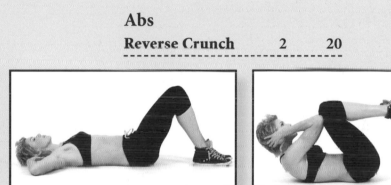

Please weigh yourself now! I bet it's quite a rush to see how much weight you've lost in such a short time. If you've reached your goal already, move on to maintenance in part 3. If not, continue training with the 10x10 Workout and of course, don't forget to stay on track with my 10x10 Diet. Hang in there. It's time to start getting more toned than you've ever been before!

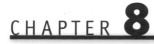

Phase 3: The Final 10 Days

The 1,500-Calorie Diet

THE THIRD TEN DAYS—you are in the final stretch! By now, *you*, not just your body, should look and feel very different. Your metabolism is turbocharged—which in turn helps your body burn fat at a faster rate. Your clothes should fit you differently. You should see muscle tone coming through and be less tired each day. Feel self-confident and strong—you've earned it. You have only ten more days left until the maintenance program.

Look in the mirror and notice how your skin and eyes are clearer. You are more radiant and I bet you've been getting compliments. Re-member that whenever possible, share with others about what you are doing and how you're feeling. People are obsessed with wellness and weight loss. You now will become the teacher and help others. You'll also receive a lot of positive reinforcement as you communicate about how you are changing your life. If you've lost more weight and inches—and I know you have—make sure you reward yourself again. Nothing increases your self-confidence more than improving your appearance and feeling confident about it. Let's get started with Phase 3, the final ten days.

Phase 3: 10 Superstar Foods

Superstar 1. Beans (kidney, black, chickpea, pinto, etc.)

Serving Size: 30g (1¼oz) cooked

Bean Facts

Calories	112
Total Fat	0g
Total Carbohydrate	20g
Fiber	6g
Protein	7g

SuperSTAR Ingredient: **Lysine**

Fat-Burning Power:

I find beans to be the best weight-loss secret in the world—thanks to lysine, an amino acid. Lysine plays a significant role in fat burning and muscle building. It works by helping the body build muscle protein, but it also has several other effects. Lysine can enhance calcium absorption and retention, which not only is important for bone health, but can also aid calcium's ability to regulate body weight. It's important for boosting growth-hormone levels as well.

Good Medicine:

- Beans are packed with soluble fiber, which dissolves in water and helps the body rid itself of cholesterol through the digestive tract.
- They balance estrogen levels in the body, especially beans such as adzuki, kidney, and pinto, and legumes like red lentils and yellow split peas.

- The lysine in beans helps in recovery from injuries, as well as assisting the body's production of hormones, enzymes, and antibodies.

Fun History:

The ancient Greeks and Romans preferred black-eyed peas.

Superstar **2. Eggs**

Serving Size: 1 large egg

Egg Facts

Calories	78
Total Fat	5.3g
Total Carbohydrate	0.6g
Fiber	0g
Protein	6.3g

SuperSTAR Ingredient: **Lecithin**

Fat-Burning Power:

I'm so passionate about eggs that the country of Australia asked me to be the spokesperson for their national egg campaign. I eat two eggs with the yolks every day of my life.

A huge part of eggs' fat-burning power lies in the fact that the yolk contains lecithin, which breaks down fat in the body. But muscle-building testosterone is synthesized from cholesterol, and as such, food containing cholesterol is a good source of building blocks for testosterone.

Eggs tame hunger with their high protein content. They also are an excellent source of omega-3 fatty acids.

Good Medicine:

- Eggs are serious brain food. The choline in eggs is also a key component of acetylcholine, a neurotransmitter in the brain that's essential for sleep, memory, attention, and mood.
- Egg yolks contain some vitamin D, which aids in calcium absorption and helps prevent osteoporosis.
- Since eggs contain all the amino acids that are needed to build keratins, a group of tough, fibrous proteins that form the structural framework of certain cells, they strengthen hair, skin, and nails.

Fun History:

Egg coloring started all the way back in the Middle Ages. While many members of the nobility and royalty exchanged eggs that were covered in gold leaf, those who were poorer dyed their eggs pretty colors and then exchanged them as gifts.

Superstar 3. Oranges

Serving Size: 1 medium orange

Orange Facts

Calories	62
Total Fat	0.1g
Total Carbohydrate	15.5g
Fiber	3.1g
Protein	1.2g

SuperSTAR Ingredient: **Vitamin C**

Fat-Burning Power:

With 95.8 milligrams of vitamin C, one orange provides 134 percent of what we need each day. Vitamin C breaks down certain amounts of cholesterol and unwanted body fats. What's more, oranges contain more than 150 different phytochemicals—and more than 60 of them are flavonoids. Flavonoids appear to act as a lipolytic agent, breaking down fat in the cells for use as fuel by the muscles.

Good Medicine:

- The flavonoids in oranges help with the treatment of vascular problems, such as varicose and spider veins. Flavonoids work by strengthening blood vessels, thus preventing these unsightly veins.
- Their high dose of vitamin A helps fight cancer.
- They help prevent forms of chronic lung disease in smokers.

Fun History:

Christopher Columbus brought the first orange seeds and seedlings to the New World on his second voyage in 1493.

Superstar **4. Peaches**

Serving Size: 1 medium peach

Peach Facts

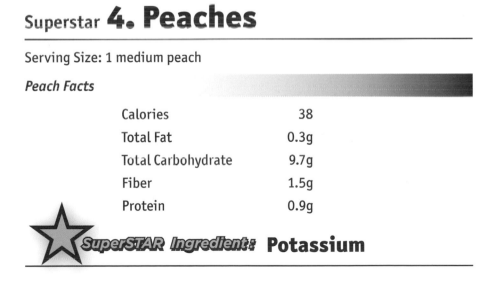

Calories	38
Total Fat	0.3g
Total Carbohydrate	9.7g
Fiber	1.5g
Protein	0.9g

SuperSTAR Ingredient: **Potassium**

Fat-Burning Power:

Potassium helps build muscles, helps muscles work properly, and helps convert the food we eat into energy. That's why it is particularly important to those of us who have weight-loss goals. Bigger muscles burn more calories, so by helping us to build slightly bigger and stronger muscles, potassium has a direct impact in helping us turn our bodies into calorie-burning machines.

Good Medicine:

- Peaches contain lots of beta-carotene to help combat the effects of aging.
- They provide a hefty helping of immune-boosting and fat-fighting vitamin C.
- And they're packed with soluble fiber for healthy digestion and for curbing sugar cravings.

Fun History:

Peaches spread to Russia and Persia (present-day Iran) probably because Chinese traders dropped peach pits along their trade routes. Alexander the Great and his armies found the peaches in Persia and brought them to Greece.

Superstar **5. Garlic**

Serving Size: 2 cloves

Garlic Facts

Calories	9
Total Fat	<0.1g
Total Carbohydrate	2g
Fiber	0.1g
Protein	0.4g

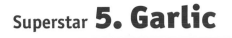 **SuperSTAR Ingredient: Allicin**

Fat-Burning Power:

Allicin burns up sugar in the body and normalizes sugar metabolism. That's good news for dieters, since excess sugar is packed away as fat. And in clinical studies, garlic can help boost testosterone while also decreasing levels of the fat-forming hormone cortisol, thus stimulating fat burning.

Good Medicine:

- Garlic can help prevent high blood pressure.
- It's used to treat diabetes.
- It lowers the risk of heart attacks.

Fun History:

Egyptians worshipped garlic and placed clay models of garlic bulbs in the tombs of pharaohs. Garlic was so highly prized, it was even used as currency.

Superstar **6. Sweet Potatoes**

Serving Size: 1 medium sweet potato

Sweet Potato Facts

Calories	103
Total Fat	0.2g
Total Carbohydrate	23.6g
Fiber	3.8g
Protein	2.3g

SuperSTAR Ingredient: **Beta-carotene**

Fat-Burning Power:

200g (7oz) of cooked sweet potatoes provides 1,922 micrograms of beta-carotene (vitamin A) if you eat it with the skin. It would take 16 cups of broccoli to provide the same amount. This is important because the beta-carotene in these potatoes helps to prevent highs and lows in blood sugar, which adds up to sustained energy throughout the day and fewer cravings. Sweet potatoes are also rich in fiber, promoting weight loss by increasing fullness and postponing hunger after meals. Despite its sweet flavor, the sweet potato is actually a slow-digesting carb that won't spike insulin levels, which would cause some of those carbs to be stored as fat.

Good Medicine:

- Sweet potatoes are high in carotenoids, which enhance muscle cell recovery after workouts.
- Their fiber combats constipation.
- They're also rich in powerful antioxidants that fight with free radicals, averting atherosclerosis, diabetic heart disease, and colon cancer.

Fun History:

Sweet potatoes are not even potatoes! In fact, they aren't even distant cousins. Sweet potatoes are part of the morning glory family (*Convolvulaceae*).

Superstar **7. Tomatoes**

Serving Size: 1 medium tomato

Tomato Facts

Calories	22
Total Fat	0.2g
Total Carbohydrate	4.8g
Fiber	1.5g
Protein	1.1g

SuperSTAR Ingredient: Biotin

Fat-Burning Power:

Tomatoes are rich in biotin, an essential water-soluble B vitamin that naturally boosts your energy. The role of biotin in the body is to help produce energy, assist in the creation of amino acids, and aid in digestion. It helps break down fats, carbohydrates, and protein into an energy source for the body both long- and short-term. Biotin also has been shown to be necessary for replication of DNA, the hereditary material in humans and almost all other organisms, and gene expression, the process by which genes turn into disease or not.

Good Medicine:

- Tomatoes are high in vitamins A and C for antioxidant protection.
- They're rich in lycopene, which has beneficial effects on IGF-1, a naturally occurring protein involved in muscle development.

- They're also high in vitamin K, which is vital for maintaining the health of your bones and regulating normal blood clotting.

Fun History:

The US Supreme Court was forced to make an official ruling as to whether this fantastic plant should be considered a vegetable or a fruit. It turns out that the tomato is both! According to the Supreme Court, the tomato is a *vegetable*; botanically, however, the tomato is a fruit.

Superstar **8. Turkey Breast**

Serving Size: 175g (6oz)

Turkey Breast Facts

Calories	230
Total Fat	1g
Total Carbohydrate	0g
Fiber	0g
Protein	51g

SuperSTAR Ingredient: **Tryptophan**

Fat-Burning Power:

Turkey is an excellent protein for weight loss. When eaten at dinner, turkey promotes the release of tryptophan, an amino acid that aids sleep. Our fat-burning hormones are released most during deep sleep. Studies show that weight gain is more prevalent in people with sleep disorders—so turkey can help sleep-related obesity.

Good Medicine:

- Turkey breast offers a generous supply of the minerals selenium and zinc for a healthy immune system.
- It has three essential B vitamins: niacin, vitamin B_6, and vitamin B_{12}, all of which help boost metabolism and promote a healthy nervous system. These vitamins also help reduce anxiety.

Fun History:

Turkey was introduced to the early Pilgrim settlers into the US by the Native American Wampanoag tribe after the Pilgrims arrived in 1620.

Superstar **9. Watercress**

Serving Size: 40g (1½oz), chopped

Watercress Facts

Calories	2
Total Fat	<0.1g
Total Carbohydrate	0.2g
Fiber	0.1g
Protein	0.4g

★ SuperSTAR Ingredient: **Glucosinolates**

Fat-Burning Power:

Watercress is rich in glucosinolates, natural compounds that increase liver detox enzymes. Watercress therefore supports liver detoxification; the liver is the metabolic factory of the entire body. The cleaner the liver, the faster your metabolism.

Good Medicine:

- Watercress acts as a diuretic to promote urine flow, thus clearing toxins from the body; its diuretic properties prevent water retention.
- Studies have shown eating watercress daily can reduce DNA damage to blood cells—damage that is considered an important trigger in the development of cancer.
- It decreases levels of triglycerides by 10 percent.

Fun History:

Watercress has been used as a medicine since ancient times to cleanse the blood and liver of toxins and enhance overall well-being. In fact, Hippocrates, the father of medicine, built his first hospital close to a watercress stream so he could use fresh sprigs to treat his patients.

Superstar 10. Yogurt, Low-Fat Greek

Serving Size: 175g (6oz)

Greek Yogurt Facts

Calories	100
Total Fat	0g
Total Carbohydrate	7g
Fiber	0g
Protein	18g

SuperSTAR Ingredient: Calcium

Fat-Burning Power:

Yogurt is rich in calcium, and that's a good thing: Calcium enhances your body's fat-burning mechanisms. The problem is that most yogurts are very high in sugar—*except* for Greek yogurt! It is more digestible than milk and thus helpful if you are lactose-intolerant (meaning you are sensitive to lactose, the sugar in milk).

Yogurt contains probiotics: live, active cultures (healthy bacteria). Scientists feel that the more of these bacteria you have, the more calories they extract from food. So you've got microscopic friends in your intestinal tract that are gobbling up excess calories and keeping them from being stored as fat.

Good Medicine:

- Greek yogurt may help prevent yeast infections, since it contains probiotics, the healthy bacteria that fight off bad material in the body.
- It improves immune response, also thanks to the action of probiotics.
- And it lowers the bad LDL cholesterol levels while increasing the good HDL.

Fun History:

In the second century, a group of nomads wandered across the Caucasus Mountains into Europe, carrying with them, among other things, goatskin bags filled with raw milk. During their travels, wild bacteria living on the bags fermented the milk inside, creating yogurt.

Phase 3: Grocery List

Produce

Several bags of salad leaves

5 medium avocados

5 bags fresh watercress

5 tins of chickpeas

5 sweet peppers

10 medium sweet potatoes

10 medium oranges

1 punnet of fresh blueberries

10 peaches

Dairy Case

20 eggs

3 x 450g (16oz) tubs of Greek yogurt

Frozen Foods

3 bags of frozen spinach

Whole Grains and Cereal

10 large wholemeal flour tortillas

Poultry

10 large turkey breasts, skinless

20 packets of low-sodium deli chicken slices

40 packets of low-sodium deli turkey slices

Other

2 packets of green tea

1 packet of herbal fruit tea

Coffee

1 packets of natural stevia leaf sweetner, such as Truvia or
Canderel Green Stevia

1 jar of minced garlic

1 bottle of olive oil

Suggested Weight-Loss Support

Whey isolate protein powder

A complete multivitamin for complete nutritional support

An omega 3–6–9 supplement for metabolic balance and beauty

QUICK PREP TIP: Boil a carton of eggs and put two each in individual ziplock bags—sprinkle with salt and pepper for a quick on the go portable snack. It's easier than cooking eggs in the morning.

Bake three sweet potatoes at once for an hour at 200°C (400°F/Gas Mark 6), or microwave separately for eight minutes each.

Microwave spinach with dash of water and garlic for one minute, 45 seconds, or steam with a splash of olive oil.

Phase 3: The Diet

Breakfast

217 calories

1 cup coffee with 1 Truvia or stevia sweetner and a dash of single cream

or

1 cup green tea

2 boiled eggs or prepared in ½ tablespoon olive oil any way you choose

1 medium orange

500ml (18fl oz) cold water

Snack

171 calories

250g (9oz) Greek yogurt sprinkled with 75g (3oz) blueberries

500ml (18fl oz) cold water

Lunch

482 calories

500ml (18fl oz) cold water

Chicken Wrap

1 large wholemeal flour tortilla

2 slices deli chicken meat

2 handfuls mixed salad leaves

½ medium avocado

25g (1oz) watercress

30g (¼oz) cooked chickpeas

½ sliced medium sweet pepper

Snack

150 calories

1 medium peach with 4 slices of low-sodium turkey deli meat

500ml (18fl oz) cold water

Dinner

1 serving (175g/6oz) turkey breast (not deli meat—baked or roasted turkey
breast without skin)

485 calories

1 medium baked sweet potato

100g (3½oz) cooked spinach with ½ tablespoon olive oil to coat pan

½ teaspoon minced garlic

500ml (18fl oz) cold water

Post-Dinner

1 cup decaf green tea with 1 bag additional herbal fruit tea

Daily Total: 1,505 calories

On the pages that follow, you'll find the Phase 3 10x10 Workout. You
will be giving it your all—but remember, you've got what it takes to succeed.

CHAPTER 9

Phase 3: The 10x10 Fitness Program

TO MAXIMIZE FAT BURNING, always keep your daily workout intensity high and add new challenges as your body adapts. That's what we'll continue to do here. At this phase, you're ready to take your intensity up a few more notches—I'm talking very high repetitions per set. High-rep training is perfect for shocking the body into progressing. I actually love this style of training and really look forward to it when it comes up on my training log.

Here's the deal: You will work three muscle groups each day with six different exercises for 100 repetitions, using the rest-pause technique to continue through each set. Perform each movement to failure (you can't lift weight again without compromising form) then rest for roughly 15 seconds and continue the movement until you reach 100 total repetitions.

Here's an overview.

Days 21, 22, and 23: You will perform six different exercises combined into one large set. You'll use the following combinations:

- chest, biceps, abs
- legs, shoulders, abs
- back, triceps, abs
- cardio-acceleration

When you lift weights, you build muscle, which is a highly meta-bolically active tissue. The higher your metabolism, the more fat you will burn. You will be supersetting most exercises. I have incorporated the proven intensity principle of cardio-acceleration on these workout days for a greater fat burn.

Day 24: You'll do interval cardio training—a fat-burning routine to help you achieve more results in less time. This is the most effective and time-efficient way to do cardio. Basically, it alternates bouts of high-intensity and lower-intensity activity. While the intense bursts burn lots of calories, the recovery periods in between draw energy straight from your fat stores, providing a two-pronged fat-burning effect.

Day 25: A full-body circuit routine. When you perform full-body workouts, you increase your fat-burning potential even more in most of your body's muscles, drawing fat into those muscles for use as energy.

Days 26, 27, and 28: You'll repeat what you did on Days 21 through 23:

- chest, biceps, abs
- legs, shoulders, abs
- back, triceps, abs
- cardio-acceleration

Day 29: Interval cardio training, just like on Day 24.
Day 30: Full-body circuit routine, just like on Day 25.

For a quick-and-easy reference chart of these exercises, please visit www.jackiewarner.com to download a chart of what you'll need to do for each day of the Phase 3 10x10 Workout.

Warm-Up Routine

Prior to every resistance-training workout for the next ten days, perform the following warm-up routine for ten reps each. You can find detailed exercise instructions in chapter 3.

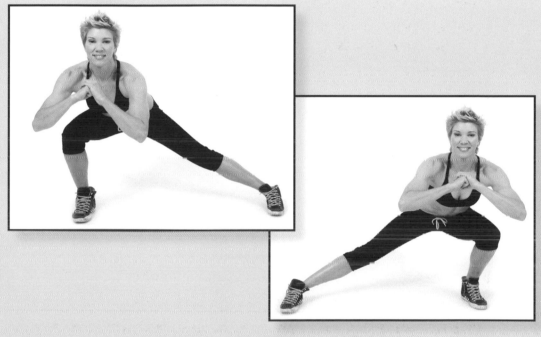

Side-to-Side Lunge

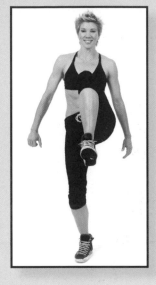

Knee-Up

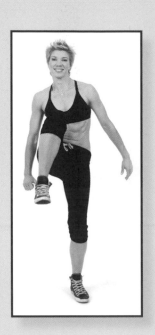

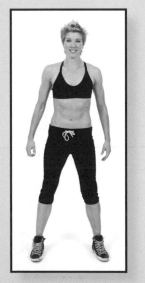

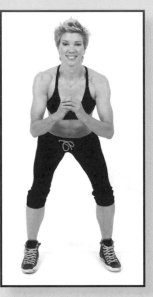

Leg Warm-Up

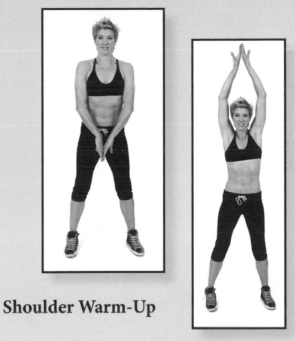

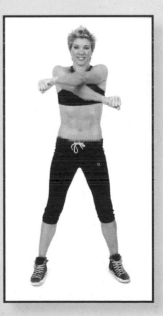

Shoulder Warm-Up

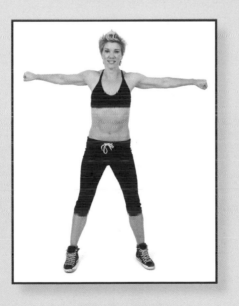

Chest Opener

Cool-Down Stretches

After every resistance-training routine for the next ten days, perform my cool-down stretches for 20 seconds each. You can find detailed exercise instructions in chapter 3.

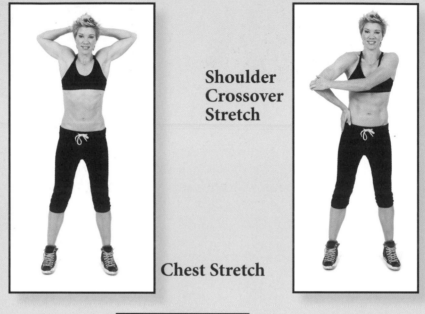

Shoulder Crossover Stretch

Chest Stretch

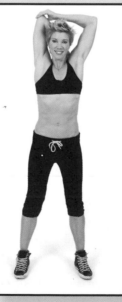

Triceps Stretch

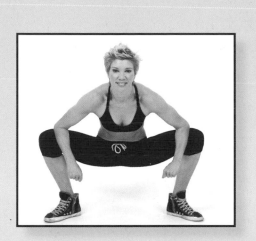

Squat Stretch

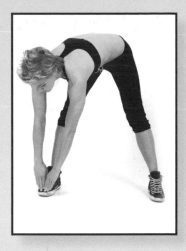

Toe Touch

DAY 21: Chest, Biceps, Abs & Cardio-Acceleration

Exercise	Sets	Reps

Chest

Flat Press	1	100

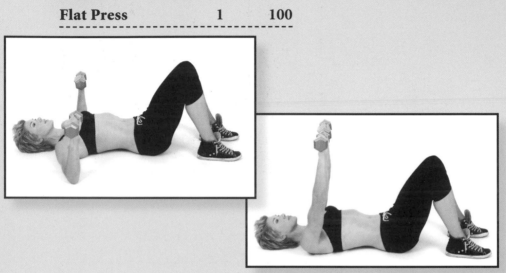

Flat Flye	1	100

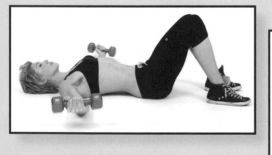
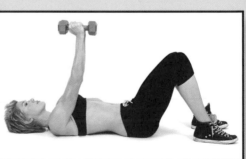

Cardio-Acceleration
200 rotations of skipping rope
1 minute rest

Biceps

Biceps Curl   1   100
- -

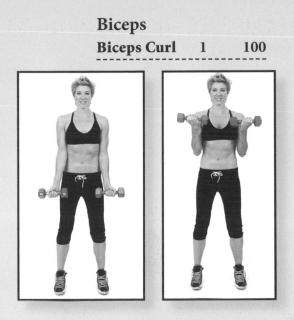

Outer Curl   1   100
- -

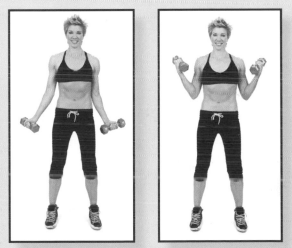

Cardio-Acceleration

200 rotations of skipping rope

1 minute rest

Abs

Reverse Crunch   1   100

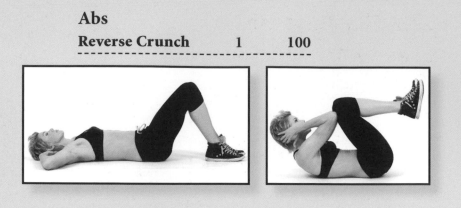

Bicycle   1   100

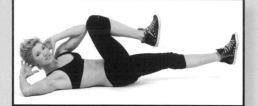 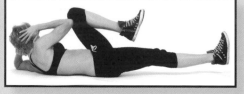

Cardio-Acceleration
200 rotations of skipping rope
1 minute rest

DAY 22: Legs, Shoulders, Abs & Cardio-Acceleration

Exercise	Sets	Reps
Legs		
Deep Squat	1	100
Sumo Squat	1	100

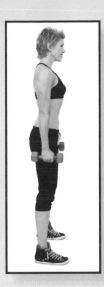

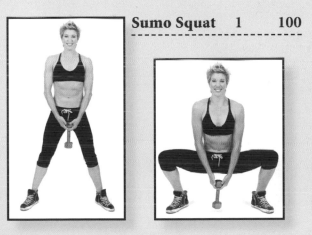

Cardio-Acceleration
200 rotations of skipping rope
1 minute rest

Shoulders

Hammer Press   1   100

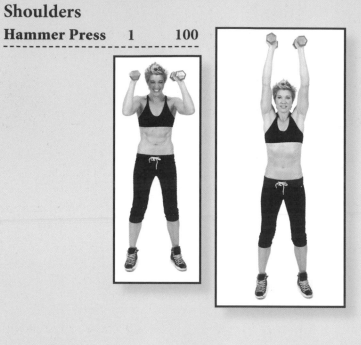

Lateral Raise   1   100

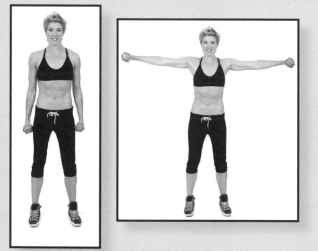

Cardio-Acceleration
200 rotations of skipping rope
1 minute rest

Abs

Up-Down Plank   1   100 total, alternating

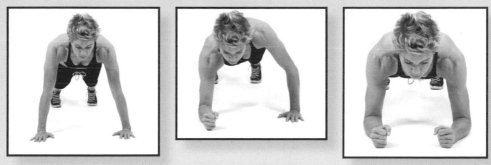

Elbow-to-Knee
Touch Plank   1   100 total, alternating

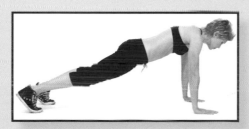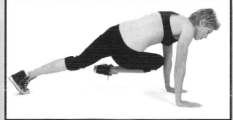

Cardio-Acceleration
200 rotations of skipping rope
1 minute rest

DAY 23: Back, Triceps, Abs & Cardio-Acceleration

Exercise	Sets	Reps

Back
Bent-Over Wide Row   1   100

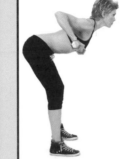

Reverse-Grip Row   1   100

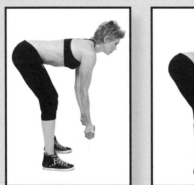
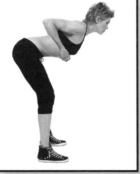

Cardio-Acceleration
200 rotations of skipping rope
1 minute rest

Triceps

Single Headbanger   1   100

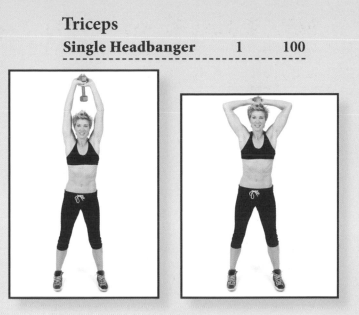

Kickback   1   100

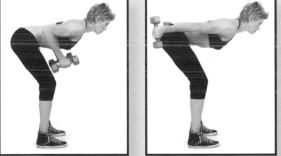

Cardio-Acceleration

200 rotations of skipping rope

1 minute rest

Abs

Straight-Leg Toe Touch   1   100

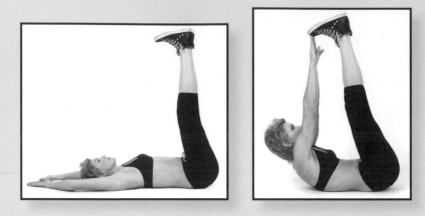

Straight-Leg Drop   1   100

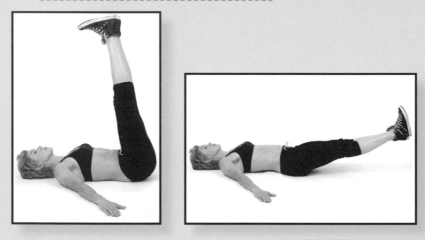

Cardio-Acceleration

200 rotations of skipping rope

1 minute rest

DAY 24: High-Intensity Interval Cardio (HIIT)

Treadmill: 3-minute treadmill jog followed by 1-minute sprint followed by 1-minute cool-down walk equaling 5 minutes. Repeat 5 more times for a total of 30 minutes.

or

Outdoor: 3-minute outdoor jog followed by 1-minute sprint followed by 1-minute cool-down walk equaling 5 minutes. Repeat 5 more times for a total of 30 minutes.

DAY 25: Full-Body Circuit

Rest only as long as it takes to get from one station to the next.

Exercise	Sets	Reps
Legs		
Sumo Squat	1	50

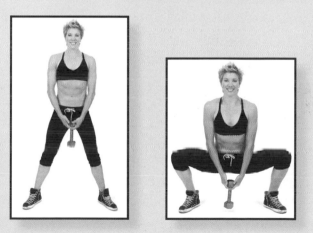

Chest
Flat Flye   1   50

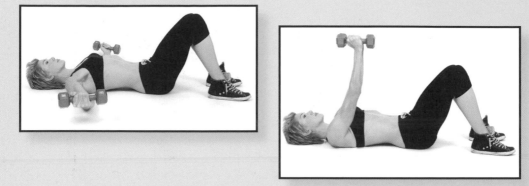

Biceps
Close Hammer Curl   1   50

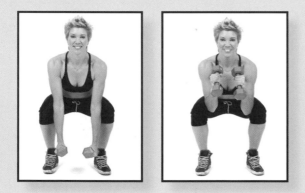

Back
Reverse-Grip Row   1   50

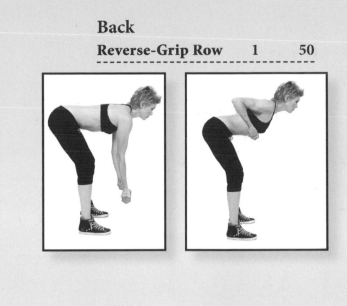

Triceps
Single Headbanger   1   50

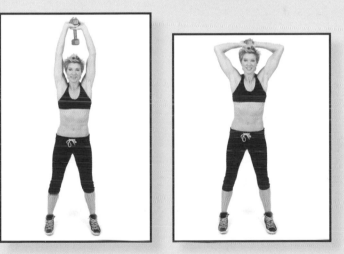

Shoulders

Lateral Raise   1   50

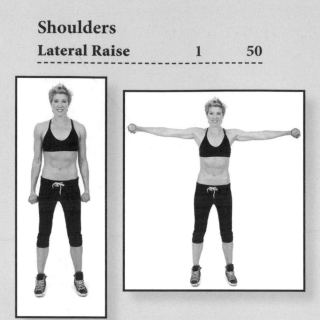

Abs

Up-Down Plank   1   50 total, alternating

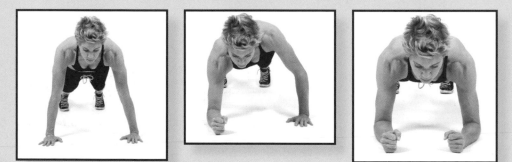

DAY 26: Chest, Biceps, Abs & Cardio-Acceleration

Exercise	Sets	Reps
Chest		
Flat Press	1	100

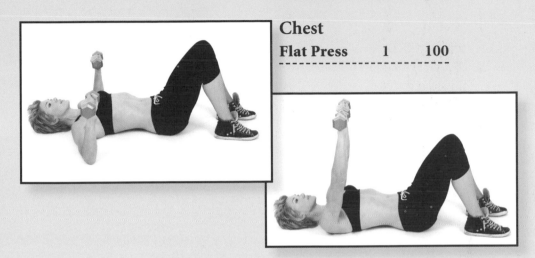

Flat Flye	1	100

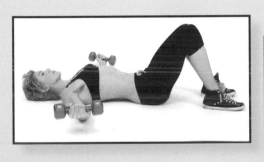
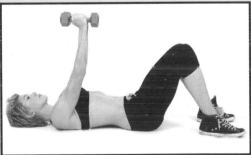

Cardio-Acceleration
200 rotations of skipping rope
1 minute rest

Biceps

Biceps Curl   1   100

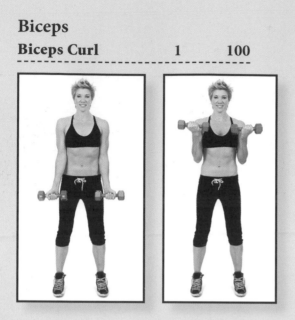

Outer Curl   1   100

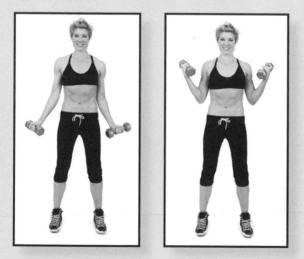

Cardio-Acceleration
200 rotations of skipping rope
1 minute rest

Abs

Reverse Crunch   1   100

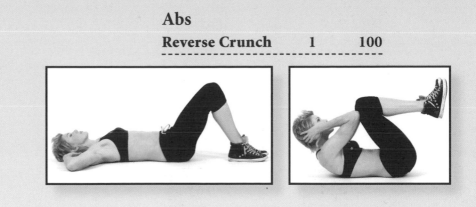

Bicycle   1   100

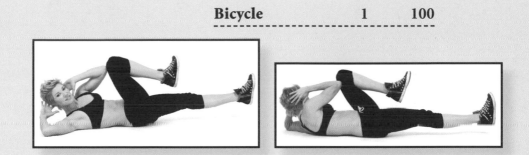

Cardio-Acceleration
200 rotations of skipping rope
1 minute rest

DAY 27: Legs, Shoulders, Abs & Cardio-Acceleration

Exercise	Sets	Reps
Legs		
Deep Squat	1	100

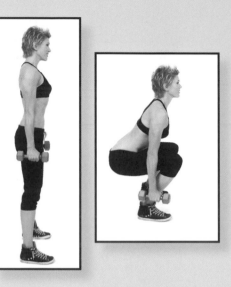

Sumo Squat	1	100

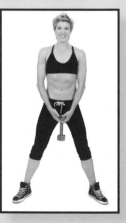
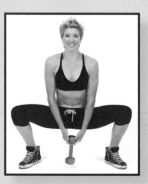

Cardio-Acceleration
200 rotations of skipping rope
1 minute rest

Shoulders

Hammer Press   1   100

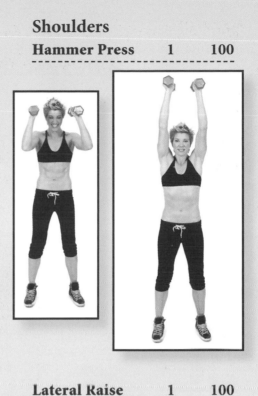

Lateral Raise   1   100

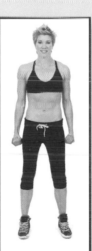

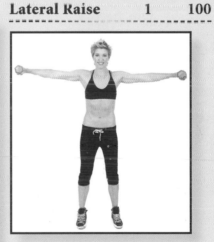

Cardio-Acceleration

200 rotations of skipping rope

1 minute rest

Abs

Up-Down Plank   1   100 total

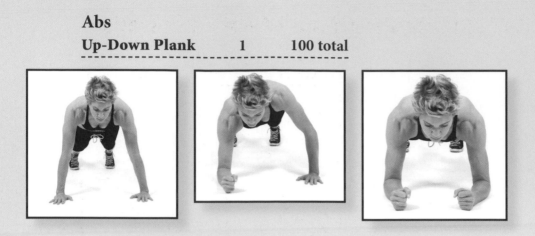

Elbow-to-Knee
Touch Plank   1   100 total , alternating

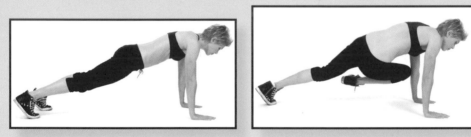

Cardio-Acceleration
200 rotations of skipping rope
1 minute rest

DAY 28: Back, Triceps, Abs & Cardio-Acceleration

Exercise	Sets	Reps

Back

Bent-Over Wide Row	1	100

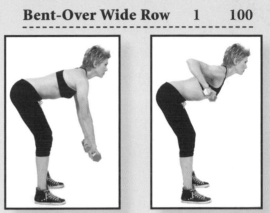

Cardio-Acceleration
200 rotations of skipping rope
1 minute rest

Back

Reverse-Grip Row	1	100

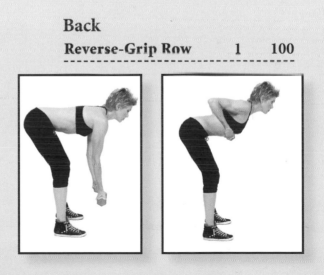

Triceps
Single Headbanger   1   100

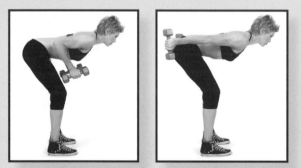

Kickback   1   100

Cardio-Acceleration
200 rotations of skipping rope
1 minute rest

Abs
Straight-Leg Toe Touch   1   100

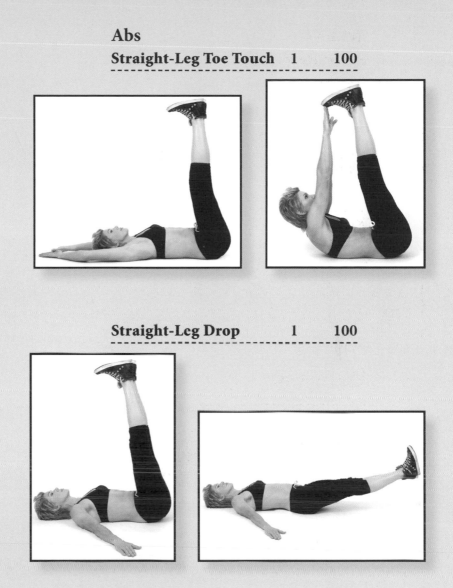

Straight-Leg Drop   1   100

Cardio-Acceleration
200 rotations of skipping rope
1 minute rest

DAY 29: High-Intensity Interval Cardio (HIIT)

Treadmill: 3-minute treadmill jog followed by 1-minute sprint followed by 1-minute cool-down walk equaling 5 minutes. Repeat 5 more times for a total of 30 minutes.

    or

Outdoor: 3-minute outdoor jog followed by 1-minute sprint followed by 1-minute cool-down walk equaling 5 minutes. Repeat 5 more times for a total of 30 minutes.

DAY 30: Full-Body Circuit

Rest only as long as it takes to get from one station to the next.

Exercise	Sets	Reps
Legs		
Sumo Squat	1	50

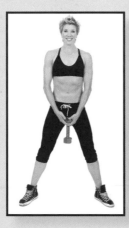 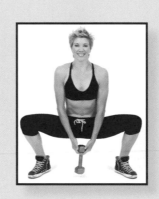

Chest
Flat Flye   1   50

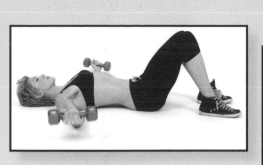

Biceps
Hammer Curl   1   50

Back
Bent-Over Wide Row 1   50

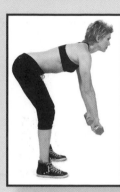
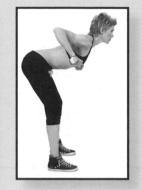

Triceps
Kickback   1   50

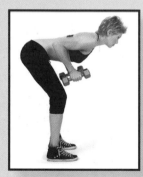
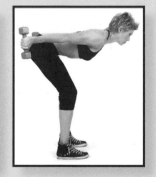

Shoulders
Lateral Raise   1   50

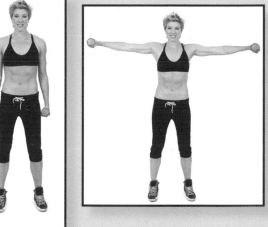

Abs
Up-Down Plank   1   50 total, alternating

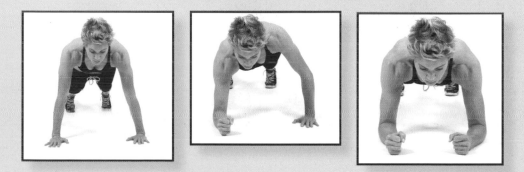

Congratulations! You've finished the 30-day program and I know you have lost a lot of weight. And I bet that's not all that has happened. You should be wearing clothes you couldn't get into a month ago because they were too small . . . buying new smaller sizes . . . and feeling optimistic about the future. I hope you have learned that you can lose weight by exercising the right way and eating simple, whole foods. You see, it wasn't that hard, was it? You didn't have to work out eight hours a day, cook elaborate meals, or pay for a trainer.

So what's next? Turn to part 3 and let me show you how to keep this beautiful new body you've got.

Keeping It Off

YOU'VE SPENT 30 DAYS eating better, feeling better, exercising better, so I know you certainly look better! The big question you're probably asking yourself is: *How can I keep this new life transformation going?*

In this section of the 10x10 Program, I'll give you the tools you need to continue your progress, whether it's additional weight loss or maintaining the weight loss you've enjoyed so far.

CHAPTER 10

Maintain Your Game!

NOW THAT YOU HAVE SUCCESSFULLY CHANGED your body and taken off that unwanted fat, it's time to eat smart for a lifetime. Take everything you have learned and apply it to your new healthy lifestyle. Nothing changes in terms of the food combinations. You should always try to eat using the food combo ratio of 45 percent carbs—35 percent protein—20 percent fat.

If you are trying to stay thin, you should eat roughly 1,500 calories per day if you are a woman and 1,800 calories per day if you are a man. If you're trying to put on muscle and gain weight, then you need to increase those calories by 300.

Maintenance Secret: Treat Meals

Here's one of the best parts of my maintenance program: You eat "clean" (healthy foods) for five days and enjoy two treat meals on the weekend. Yes, you get to "cheat" for *two* meals! After working with countless clients, I found that one treat meal a week was not enough to stay on track long-term. Clients felt literally cheated out of one of life's greatest pleasures, and they started slipping up all through the week. Not until I added the second treat meal did everyone start responding in phenomenal ways. So during the week, you'll eat like you're at work, knowing the light's at the end of the tunnel.

Rules for Treat Meals

- Treat meals should be less than 1,500 calories each.
- You must be working out to intensity five times a week.
- Plan your treat meals in advance.
- Throw treat leftovers away.
- If you drink, make alcohol a treat meal. And if you drink every day, reduce from two drinks a day to one.

Examples of treat meals include:

- Dinner with friends, in which you eat what you want, including drinks and dessert (1,200–1,500 calories)
- Sweets (140g/5oz packet of peanut M&M's) and a medium pop-corn at the movies (1,100 calories)
- A Sunday-morning brunch—eggs Benedict, ham, and tomatoes (780 calories)

I treat myself to all these foods, guilt-free, knowing that on Monday I resume my five days of clean eating. Because I haven't said no to myself, I am happy and not deprived.

With treat meals, you have structure and flexibility with a way to get thin that feels good. This is the only way of eating that works in my life and the lives of countless others. This is a lifestyle and not a diet. What is amazing about eating clean for five days is that you break your addiction to sugar and you kill cravings so that you don't even want as much on your treat meal days.

My Maintenance Plan Overview

Remember, simple, simple, simple. Follow these daily guidelines and just plug in foods from my list:

- Each day, eat five meals a day: breakfast, lunch, and dinner, plus a midmorning and midafternoon snack.
- Each day, choose four proteins, three vegetables, two fruits, two grains, and one fat from my list of foods. (See "Maintenance Foods," p. 276.)
- Add veggies to two of your meals plus one snack or to a whey isolate protein powder shake.
- Eat one snack or meal daily with a clean fat, such as avocado, nuts, seeds, or flaxseed oil.
- Eat low-fat dairy foods (including hard cheeses) sparingly—no more than one serving a day (preferably cottage cheese). And: No milk.
- Eat two servings of fresh fruit daily. Enjoy them with meals or as snacks, and try to combine them with some protein.
- Eat a variety of foods each week. Rotate your fruits, veggies, and protein selections frequently.
- Drink three liters of water daily.
- Enjoy two treat meals on the weekend.

Maintenance Foods

To keep your weight off, here's what else you get to eat. You'll simply choose foods from the following categories each day. Remember to go to the Superstar Foods I've highlighted in each phase of the 10x10 Program. These foods will give you the most nutrition per serving and offer other health benefits as well. The Superstar Foods are identified with a star to help you make fast-and-easy food decisions.

Proteins—Eat Four 115g (4oz) Servings a Day

FISH AND SHELLFISH:

Clams

Cod

Flounder

Haddock

Halibut

Lobster

Monkfish

Oysters

Perch

Pollack

Red snapper

Salmon, wild ☆

Sardines, water-packed

Scallops

Shrimp

Sole

Tilapia

Trout

Whitefish

LEAN POULTRY (CHICKEN AND TURKEY):

Chicken breasts, skinless ☆

Guinea fowl, skinless

Turkey breasts, skinless ☆

LEAN MEAT:

Flank steak

Sirloin

Tenderloin

Pork tenderloin

Pork rib chops

Pork roast

Lamb roast

Lamb chops

Leg of lamb

LOW-FAT DAIRY FOODS:

(Limit these to up to two of your
    protein servings per day)
Greek-style low-fat yogurt ☆
Low-calorie cheeses (Brie,
    Camembert, Fontina, low-fat
    Cheddar, Edam, feta, goat's
    cheese, and part-skim
    mozzarella)
Low-fat cottage cheese ☆
Low-fat ricotta cheese
Whey powder ☆
Eggs (eat two eggs each day) ☆

BEANS AND LEGUMES (60G /2¼ OZ = 1 PROTEIN SERVING):

Adzuki beans
Bean soups
Black beans ☆
Black-eyed peas
Broad beans
Chickpeas ☆
Haricot beans
Kidney beans ☆
Lentils
Lentil soups
Lima beans

Navy beans
Pinto beans ☆
Red beans
Split peas
Soybeans
White beans

Vegetables—Eat 3 Portions a Day

Alfalfa sprouts ☆
Artichokes
Artichoke hearts
Asparagus ☆
Aubergine
Beetroot
Beet greens
Broccoli ☆
Broccoli sprouts
Brussels sprouts
Cabbage
Carrots ☆
Cauliflower
Celery ☆
Chilis
Coriander
Courgettes

Cucumbers

Endive

Fennel

Garlic

Green beans

Kale

Kelp and other edible seaweeds

Leeks

Lettuce, all varieties

Mangetout

Mushrooms

Mustard greens

Okra

Onions ☆

Parsley

Parsnips

Peas

Peppers, all varieties

Potatoes (new)

Pumpkin

Radishes

Rhubarb

Spinach ☆

Spring greens

Spring onions

Summer squash

Swede

Sweetcorn

Sweet peppers (red) ☆

Sweet potatoes ☆

Swiss chard

Tomatoes ☆

Turnips

Turnip greens

Watercress ☆

Winter squash (acorn, butternut, etc.)

Yams

Fruits—Eat 2 Whole Fruits or 2 Portions of Chopped Fresh Fruit a Day

Apricots

Bananas, underripe

Blackberries

Blueberries ☆

Cantaloupe

Cherries

Cranberries

Currants

Dates

Figs

Grapes

Kiwi

Kumquats

Grapefruit ☆

Guava

Honeydew melon

Lemons

Limes

Mangoes

Oranges ☆

Papayas

Pears

Peaches ☆

Pineapples

Plums

Pomegranates

Prunes

Raisins

Raspberries

Strawberries

Tangerines

Tangelos

Watermelons

Grains—Eat 2 x 250g (9oz) Servings a Day or 2 Slices (unless otherwise specified)

Barley

Bran (15g/½oz = 1 serving)

Brown rice ☆

Buckwheat

Bulgur wheat

Cornmeal

Millet

Oats

Oat bran

Porridge ☆

Quinoa

Rye

Spelt

Wheat germ (15g/½oz = 1 serving)

Wholemeal products (dark nutty breads, crackers, pita bread, tortillas, etc.) (1 piece or slice = 1 serving)

Wholemeal or vegetable pastas (100g/3½oz = 1 serving)

Fat Selections—Eat 2 Tablespoons a Day (unless otherwise specified)

Almonds

Almond butter (raw)

Avocado (¼ fruit = 1 serving fat) ☆

Butter

Brazil nuts

Flaxseeds

Flaxseed oil

Hazelnuts

Olive oil

Pecans

Pine nuts

Walnuts

Walnut oil

Peanut butter (sugar-free, all natural) ☆

Pumpkin seeds

Sesame seeds

Sunflower seeds

Creating Maintenance Meals

Using the food selection guidelines I've outlined, your three meals and two snacks each day will include four proteins, three vegetables, two fruits, two grains, and one fat. And don't forget to drink three liters of water a day.

Maintenance Menus

I've included three days' worth of sample menus to help you get started on your maintenance plan. These daily meals add up to roughly 1,500 calories.

Day 1

Breakfast

1 cup coffee with 1 Truvia or stevia sweetner and a dash of almond milk

or

1 cup green tea

75g (3oz) porridge with 25g (1oz) blueberries and 4 walnuts, sweetened with Truvia or stevia sweetner and cinnamon

500ml (18fl oz) cold water

Snack

1 medium apple with 125g (4½oz) cottage cheese

500ml (18fl oz) cold water

Lunch

Dark green leafy salad with sweet red peppers, onion, 2 tomato slices,
and ¼ avocado
1 chicken breast
1 slice toasted wholemeal bread
500ml (18fl oz) cold water

Snack

½ sliced cucumber with 3 tablespoons hummus
500ml (18fl oz) cold water

Dinner

Salmon fillet with garlic, 250g (9oz) quinoa, and 175g (6oz) broccoli
500ml (18fl oz) cold water

Post-Dinner

1 bag decaf green tea with 1 bag fruity tea

Day 2

Breakfast

2 low-fat wholemeal tortillas, each filled with 1 scrambled egg and
1 tablespoon salsa
500ml (18fl oz) cold water

Snack

8 grapes with 6 almonds
500ml (18fl oz) cold water

Lunch

Dark green leafy salad with sweet red peppers, onion, 2 tomato slices,
and ¼ avocado
1 chicken breast
500ml (18fl oz) cold water

Snack

115g (4oz) low-fat cottage cheese with ½ banana
500ml (18fl oz) cold water

Dinner

115g (4oz) pork tenderloin with 175g (6oz) steamed broccoli and 1 baked
sweet potato
500ml (18fl oz) cold water

Post-Dinner

1 bag decaf green tea mixed with 1 bag favorite herbal tea

Day 3

Breakfast

Jackie's Breakfast Smoothie

1 teaspoon sugar-free, all-natural peanut butter

75g (2½oz) plain instant porridge (uncooked)

25g (1oz) mixed frozen berries

25g (1oz) frozen spinach

1 scoop whey isolate protein powder

Dash of water

500ml (18fl oz) cold water

Snack

225g (8oz) low-fat cottage cheese with 25g (1oz) blueberries and 4 walnuts
500ml (18fl oz) cold water

Lunch

1 pan-grilled salmon fillet prepared with 1 tablespoon lemon juice and
½ teaspoon dill in ½ tablespoon olive oil or pre-prepared from deli section
of grocery

5 frozen asparagus stalks, steamed or microwaved

100g (3½oz) wild rice (preferably instant) prepared with salt and pepper

500ml (18fl oz) cold water

Snack

2 boiled eggs

500ml (18fl oz) cold water

Dinner

115g (4oz) grilled chicken with 1 cup asparagus

200g (7oz) chopped fresh pineapple

500ml (18fl oz) cold water

Post-Dinner

1 bag decaf green tea mixed with 1 bag favorite herbal tea

Maintain Your Muscle!

I have given you different plateau-preventing techniques that you can use forever to maintain the new tone that I know you have. Remember that you need to change training styles or increase weight resistance in order to prevent plateaus. Here are all the exercises that you can use forever. Be creative in how you combine them. For example, you can use the same exercises but try a different combination.

This is called a five-day split. You can add two days of rest nonconsecutively in this week. Throw these in your existing routines for amazing, continued results!

Here are examples:

- Work only the chest one day, combining all chest exercises with four cardio-accelerations (200 rotations each).
- Work only the back one day, using all back exercises with four cardio-accelerations (200 rotations each).
- Work only the legs one day, using all leg exercises with four cardio-accelerations (200 rotations each).
- Work only the biceps and triceps one day, using all arm exercises with cardio-acceleration (200 rotations each).
- Work only the shoulders and abs one day, using all shoulder and ab exercises with cardio-acceleration (200 rotations each).

Have fun with your combinations and change every month for continued success. Go online to www.jackiewarner.com to download a ton more exercises and plateau busters.

Chest

Flat Press

Incline Press

Flat Flye

Push-Up

Back

Bent-Over Wide Row

Reverse-Grip Row

Alternating Row

Rear Lateral Raise

Legs

Deep Squat

Deadlift

Sumo Squat

Front Alternating
   Lunge

Biceps

Biceps Curl

Close Hammer Curl

Diagonal Curl

Outer Curl

Triceps

Close-Grip Press

Single Headbanger

Kickback

Standing Alternating
   Extension

Shoulders

Military Press

Hammer Press

Lateral Raise

Front Raise

Abs

Bicycle

Reverse Crunch

Elbow-to-Knee Touch Plank

Up-Down Plank

Straight-Leg Toe Touch

Straight-Leg Drop

Journal It

With my program, you don't need to keep a food journal, because it's all there for you. But I do recommend keeping a workout training log during your maintenance program. I still carry my little book into the gym every day. Transfer your exercises into your log; then if you don't feel sore from them, you know that your weight is not heavy enough or you're not following the rules of the routine. Keep track of your goals in a training journal, too. Evaluate your progress regularly. It's an absolute must to track your reps, sets, and increases with resistance training. Over time, your written log will help you identify strengths, weaknesses, and improvements in your physique. Seeing your progress on paper is incredibly motivating. You'll be encouraged and inspired when you look back on your entries and see how far you've come.

In your training log, be sure to note any significant feelings, mental or physical, that occur in response to working out. If I'm not sore after my back routine, for example, I make a note of this. This feedback tells me I need to change weight or exercise groupings. On the other hand, put a smiley face next to the days when working out made you feel sore. Soreness means great things are happening to your muscles. Keeping tabs on your progress (or lack thereof) is the only way to accurately assess your workouts, stay accountable, and devise solutions to problems.

CHAPTER **11**

Top Tips

COMPLETING THE 10X10 PROGRAM is the first step to a healthier, happier life. Now you are going back out into the world, and you may need some additional help from time to time.

The useful tips here are one way to continue on your fitness journey. Even if you take one or two from each section, you'll notice big changes. Another is to visit my website regularly at www.jackiewarner.com for the latest in nutrition, exercise, mental strategies, and community support.

TIP1   BOOST "WEIGHT-LOSS" HORMONES

(HGH, TESTOSTERONE, PROGESTERONE)

❏ Cut back on carbs at night. This will help keep your blood sugar levels down and increase your HGH.

❏ Get a good night's sleep (deep sleep leads to high HGH production).

❏ Eat foods high in vitamin B and zinc, including whole grains, legumes, vegetables, and proteins.

❏ Eat organic foods when possible.

❏ Exercise regularly.

❏ Eat foods rich in beta-carotene, such as yellow and orange veggies, and green leafy vegetables.

❏ Consume foods high in B vitamins, boron, and foods high in amino acids such as whole grains and meats.

❏ Watch your fat intake (limit red meat to three servings a week). Eat more poultry and fish, and avoid fatty meats such as those found in deep-fried, smoked, or salt-cured foods.

❏ Watch your caffeine and alcohol intake.

TIP2 | FIGHT "FAT" HORMONES
(INSULIN, ESTROGEN, CORTISOL, GHRELIN)

☐ Add whole foods such as porridge in place of processed and high-sugar foods.

☐ Enjoy fruit often; it's the best defense against insulin spikes.

☐ Be prepared to combat cravings. Stash healthy snacks in your handbag, desk, or car.

☐ Stay away from high-protein diets; they cause serotonin levels to fall and create sugar cravings.

☐ Move your body. Working out helps reduce cravings. If you feel a craving coming on, immediately step outside for a walk, take the stairs, or hop on the treadmill.

☐ Eliminate sugar and processed foods from your diet, and consume hormone-free meat, eggs, and dairy. (Use good natural sweeteners like Truvia or Canderel Green Stevia.)

☐ Eat foods high in fiber.

☐ Reduce alcohol and caffeine intake (drink no more than two cups of coffee a day).

☐ Don't eat out of heated plastic containers (they can release BPA, which produces estrogen).

☐ Keep stress in check (stress decreases progesterone and raises cortisol levels, which reduces testosterone).

☐ Keep cortisol levels in check by eating regular healthy meals that include foods high in casein like cottage cheese, green

TIP2 CONT'D

vegetables, whole-grain breads, mushrooms, and fruits, especially berries.

☐ Ease back on foods high in MSG (Asian food, for example).

☐ Get enough rest.

☐ Eat fish.

☐ Eat slowly (it takes at least 20 minutes for leptin, the hormone that tells your body it's full, to kick in after a meal).

☐ Take zinc.

☐ Drink two to three liters of water a day.

☐ Eliminate fried and processed foods (they interfere with blood circulation and lymphatic drainage).

☐ Eat cellulite-busting vegetables such as kale, broccoli, brussels sprouts, parsley, green pepper, asparagus (a great diuretic), and root veggies.

☐ Eat apples.

☐ Exercise regularly to increase lymph flow.

TIP3 CUT OUT BAD SUGARS

Any three of the following tips not only kill sugar cravings, but help boost weight loss as well.

- ☐ Eat foods that contain less than five grams of sugar.
- ☐ Eliminate sugar-free juices, fizzy drinks, or treats; they cause sugar cravings.
- ☐ Don't put sugar in clean beverages such as coffee, tea, or water.
- ☐ Remove simple sugar items from your home.
- ☐ Throw away leftover treat meals.
- ☐ Buy apples, pears, berries, and citrus fruits instead of processed sugar snacks.
- ☐ Use Truvia or a stevia sweetner instead of sugar.
- ☐ Exercise regularly (20 minutes of rigorous physical activity brings a rush of endorphins); schedule lunch workouts.
- ☐ Drink lots of water (cravings are usually due to dehydration, not hunger).
- ☐ Cut back on caffeine.
- ☐ Eat sugar-free foods, not fat-free foods.

TIP4 CLEAN UP YOUR ORGANS

Healthy organs turn your body into a fat-burning machine.

- [ ] Eat detox foods daily, such as apricots, artichokes, beetroot, blueberries, and green leafy vegetables.
- [ ] Drink two to three liters of water a day.
- [ ] Eat organic food whenever possible.
- [ ] Increase fiber intake to 25 to 35 grams a day by eating high-fiber foods like fruits, veggies, and whole grains.
- [ ] Add whey powder to your diet—it's beneficial to muscles, the cardiovascular system, and other vital organs.
- [ ] Eliminate excessive amounts of milk and dairy.
- [ ] Eat vitamin C and magnesium-rich foods.
- [ ] Exercise regularly.
- [ ] Eliminate refined carbs and sugars.
- [ ] Eliminate or reduce acetaminophen products like paracetamol.
- [ ] Reduce prescription drug use—don't work against the body's delicate balancing system with meds unless necessary. Think less medication, more motivation.
- [ ] Avoid fatty meats (salt-cured, smoked, deep-fried).
- [ ] Eliminate or reduce consumption of fluoride in tap water. (Fluoride blocks iodine receptors in the thyroid glands, halts hormone production, and can contribute to hypothyroidism.)

| TIP5 | # ADD THESE SUPERSTAR FOODS EVERY DAY |

☐ Eat two eggs a day. Eggs are a great fat-burning food; they contain lecithin, which curbs the appetite.

☐ Eat one serving of porridge a day (fat burner). It's one of the healthy carbs. It's slow digesting and kills cravings. It also keeps insulin levels steady. Keep packets of instant porridge handy in your handbag or in your desk or locker at work.

☐ Eat two to three servings of hormone-balancing detox veggies a day. They are natural fat burners and are loaded with fiber (page 277 has lots of examples). Sneak veggies into regular meals—for example, by putting spinach into a fruit shake. You'll mask the taste and get the nutrients.

☐ Eat two servings of fruit a day (two whole fruits). They digest slowly and help with weight loss.

☐ Eat whole fruit instead of drinking juice.

☐ Drink two to three liters of water a day, including one bottle of water with your morning coffee.

☐ Satisfy oral fixations and cravings by drinking one teabag of decaf green tea with one teabag of herbal fruit tea every night.

TIP6 SUBSTITUTE GOOD FATS FOR BAD FATS

☐ Prepare food by roasting, baking, griddling, steaming, and grilling without added fat.

☐ Use olive oil cooking spray.

☐ Remove skin and fat from meat prior to cooking.

☐ Make your own salad dressing with oil and balsamic vinegar.

☐ Use sugar-free, all-natural peanut butter or raw almond butter instead of butter on toast.

☐ Use more seasoning and less butter.

☐ Use low-fat condiments.

☐ Cook with lean ground turkey instead of ground beef.

TIP7 LEARN HOW TO EAT AT A RESTAURANT

- ☐ Eat the good, the bad, and the ugly in that order on your plate.
- ☐ Call ahead and get the menu.
- ☐ Ask the waiter to hold the bread.
- ☐ If you're eating clean, order a meat main course with vegetables and a salad.
- ☐ Order sauces and dressings on the side.
- ☐ Be assertive. Ask about preparation methods.
- ☐ Don't eat foods that are fried, sautéed, or cooked in heavy cream.
- ☐ Practice portion control.

TIP8 CREATE AN ENVIRONMENT OF WELLNESS

☐ Clean house. Remove all junk food and trigger food.

☐ Use smaller-sized dishes.

☐ Don't eat in front of the television.

☐ When you're grocery shopping, shop the perimeter first—outside in.

☐ Variety is the spice of life. Try a new food each week to prevent boredom.

☐ Enlist support. Get loved ones involved in your cause. Ask for what you need in terms of support that doesn't put others on the defensive.

TIP9   MAKE WORKOUTS FUN AND EASY

☐ Exercise with intensity (this means pushing yourself for shorter periods of time) and consistency five days a week.

☐ "It's not how long; it's how strong." Shorten your cardio and always apply HIIT.

☐ Muscle is the quickest way to a healthy body. It helps speed up metabolism so that you can burn calories while resting.

☐ Exercise at a time of day when you are most energized.

☐ Schedule an appointment with a trainer or class to keep you on track.

☐ Circuit training simultaneously improves mobility, strength, and stamina, and is the best way to burn calories the fastest.

☐ Change your routine so the body keeps changing. Avoid plateaus at all costs.

☐ Reduce rest times between sets. This will increase your production of HGH.

☐ Evaluate your progress regularly. Keep a training log. Put smiley faces next to sore days. Take your before measurements, then wait one month and take your after measurements.

TIP10

STAY POSITIVE WITH THESE MENTAL EXERCISES

Attitude is everything! Think of food and exercise as powerful medicine. Love the burn and the sweat. Equate them with results. See a diet as an exciting new adventure and a way to make your body beautiful.

Set realistic goals. Make goals athletic and performance-based. These are quantifiable. Make a list of everything you can do to achieve your goals, including the reasons why you don't want to be fat and why you want to be thin, and carry it with you at all times. Talk about your goals with friends and family. It helps your goals become reality.

Visualization is a powerful tool. "See" the muscles working as you move through exercises. Visualize yourself at your dream weight, in a swimsuit having childlike fun at the pool. Visualize confidently flirting or finding inner sexiness. See yourself exercising and loving it. Visualize yourself doing a whole set without tiring.

Negative attracts negative. If you are negative about yourself, you will attract failure. If you catch yourself thinking negatively, say your name out loud and say the word "*Stop*." Then rephrase the statement in a positive way. See yourself as an athlete. Behavior is consistent with identity. If you identify with physical activity, you'll make it part of your lifestyle.

You move toward what you focus on. See yourself getting healthier. Don't just hope to lose the weight; assume you will lose it. Focus on being fit and how strong you're getting, how well you're sleeping, and how happy you are. Look at yourself in the mirror. See what you want to see, and you will become it.

Listen to your favorite music while working out. It will link the workout to pleasure and inspire movement.

Don't overthink it. Just do it.

Bonus Blogs

I've had the privilege of blogging for some of the country's most respected websites and media outlets. A complete library of my blog posts is available at my website, www.jackiewarner.com. You might find them helpful as you continue to weave the 10x10 Program into your life.

Welcome to Your New Life!

If you've reached this part of the book, then I know you've had a life-changing month. Using the 10x10 Program, you've learned how to eat healthier, you've set a pattern for daily workouts, and your self-esteem is blowing the roof off the house!

Trust me. I know the feeling.

We must walk through our fears in order to make it to the other side, the side that gives us freedom, that empowers us, and that ultimately gives us the life and body we have always wanted.

It all comes down to three things:

√ **Eat**

√ **Move**

√ **Believe**

We have to *eat* whole and nutritious foods.

We are built to *move* our bodies. There are no easier ways.

We have to *believe* that we deserve to be healthy and happy. We have the freedom to choose our own destiny.

I have committed myself and my life to helping you achieve the body and life you deserve. And now I challenge *you* to take all that you have learned and empower the people around you to change their lives.

Jackie Warner

References

Ahtiainen, J. P., and Häkkinen, K. 2009. Strength athletes are capable to produce greater muscle activation and neural fatigue during high-intensity resistance exercise than nonathletes. *Journal of Strength and Conditioning Research* 23:1129–1134.

Anderson, J. W., et al. 1999. Long-term weight maintenance after an intensive weight-loss program. *Journal of the American College of Nutrition* 18:620–627.

Davis, W. J. 2008. Concurrent training enhances athletes' strength, muscle endurance, and other measures. *Journal of Strength and Conditioning Research* 22:1487–1502.

Depcik, E., et al. 2004. Weight training and body satisfaction of body-image-disturbed college women. *Journal of Applied Sport Psychology* 16:287–299.

Editor. 2011. Sleep less, eat more: study; those who slept 4 hours consumed about 300 more calories a day than those who slept 9 hours. *Consumer Health News*. Online, March 23.

Forman, A. 2001. Milk wars: is the growing backlash against "Bessie" justified? *Environmental Nutrition*. Online.

Grand, R. J., and Montgomery, R. K. 2008. Lactose malabsorption. *Current Treatment Options in Gastroenterology* 11:19–25.

Larsson, S. C., et al. 2006. Milk, milk products and lactose intake and ovarian cancer risk: a meta-analysis of epidemiological studies. *International Journal of Cancer* 118:431–441.

Meijerink, M., et al. 2010. Identification of genetic loci in *Lactobacillus plantarum* that modulate the immune response of dendritic cells using comparative genome hybridization. *PLoS One* 13:5:e10632.

Nackers, L. M., et al. 2010. The association between rate of initial weight loss and long-term success in obesity treatment: does slow and steady win the race? *International Journal of Behavioral Medicine* 17:161–167.

Outwater, J. L., et al. 1997. Dairy products and breast cancer: the IGF-1, estrogen, and bGH hypothesis. *Medical Hypotheses* 48:453–461.

Rock, C. L. 2011. Milk and the risk and progression of cancer. *Nestlé Nutrition Workshop Series* 67:173–185.

Stallknecht, B., et al. 2007. Are blood flow and lipolysis in subcutaneous adipose tissue influenced by contractions in adjacent muscles in humans? *American Journal of Physiology, Endocrinology, and Metabolism* 292(2):E394–399.

Willoughby, D. S., et al. 2007. Effects of resistance training and protein plus amino acid supplementation on muscle anabolism, mass, and strength. *Amino Acids* 32:467–477.

Index

About the Author

A Midwestern girl turned self-made millionaire at the age of 22, Jackie was inspired to pursue a career in fitness and nutrition after training a few close friends with dramatic life-changing results. Within a year, Jackie opened her first health center, Lift. The revolutionary fitness facility was the first health club in Southern California to accept health insurance for exercise.

From 2004 to 2009, Jackie owned and operated her next gym, Sky Sport & Spa. Employing Jackie's complete approach to fitness, Sky Sport was the nation's premiere full service health and medical practice. Although frequented by fitness aficionados for years, Sky Sport was introduced to the rest of the world on Jackie's hit television show, *Work Out*.

She returned to television in 2010 in the Bravo show, *Thintervention with Jackie Warner*. Hailed by critics, the premiere gave the network its best ratings ever for a Monday.

Jackie is one of the world's most sought-after fitness experts by media and consumers alike. She is a regular contributor to *The Huffington Post, Fitness Rx,* and *Fitness* magazine, and she wrote the *New York Times* bestseller, *This is Why You're Fat (and How to Get Thin Forever)*, and stars in several best-selling DVDs.

Jackie is the current face of a health and wellness campaign called Fit in Your Skin, and is the national spokesperson for Eggs of Australia.

To help people take back further control of their lives, Jackie is creating a new online community and product line set to launch in early 2012. This new program will provide workouts; healthy recipes; and fitness, nutrition, and lifestyle tips.

To learn more, please visit **www.jackiewarner.com**.